Natural Solutions
to Infertility

About The Author

For over 20 years, Dr Marilyn Glenville has practised nutrition in the UK and USA. She specialises in the natural approach to female hormone problems and runs clinics in London and Kent. She is one of the UK's leading experts in nutritional health for women.

As a respected authority on women's healthcare, Dr Glenville gives regular talks on radio and has often appeared on television and in the press. She frequently advises health professionals and lectures at academic conferences held at the Medical Society and the Royal College of Physicians. She obtained her doctorate from Cambridge University and is a Fellow of the Royal Society of Medicine and a member of the Nutrition Society. Dr Glenville has been officially appointed by the Foods Standards Agency to be an observer on the Expert Group on the safety of Vitamins and Minerals. She is also a steering group member of the Forum on Food and Health at the Royal Society of Medicine.

Dr Glenville's previous books include the bestselling *Natural Solutions to Infertility, Nutritional Health Handbook* (both Piatkus), *Natural Alternatives to HRT* and *Natural Alternatives to Dieting*.

Natural Solutions to Infertility

How to increase your chances of conceiving and preventing miscarriage

Marilyn Glenville PhD

PIATKUS

To my children – Matthew, Leonard and Chantell

Copyright © 2000 by Marilyn Glenville

Published in the UK in 2000 by
Judy Piatkus (Publishers) Limited
5 Windmill Street
London W1T 2JA
e-mail: info@piatkus.co.uk

Reprinted 2001, 2002 (twice), 2003, 2004, 2005

For the latest news and information on all our titles,
visit our website at www.piatkus.co.uk

The moral rights of the author have been asserted

A catalogue record for this book is available from the British Library

ISBN 0 7499 2059 9

Page design by Paul Saunders
Edited by Kelly Davis

Typeset by Phoenix Photosetting, Chatham, Kent
Printed and bound in Great Britain
by CPI Bath Press

Contents

Foreword

I am very pleased to write a foreword for this book because I know that there are many natural alternatives to help couples achieve fertility and I share the approach and the sentiments expressed in the book.

Marilyn has a comprehensive and practical grasp of nutrition and other complementary approaches to fertility. She practises the concept of 'Integrated Healthcare' which I believe is the way forward for the new millennium. This approach provides the best of conventional 'high-tech' medical care combined with the many benefits that the world of complementary medicine has to offer.

My own gynaecology and fertility practice is based on the same holistic approach. Recent advances now allow a couple to be investigated with a minimum of invasive testing. Information which previously would have only been available by laparoscopy is now easily obtained by a simple ultrasound scan and blood tests. The investigation for both partners can be collated within one menstrual cycle – without the use of any operative procedures.

I agree with Marilyn's emphasis on the importance of nutrition and lifestyle to help a couple conceive and give birth. Lifestyle changes also have a very significant knock-on effect later in life and both partners will have a reduced risk of cancer, heart attacks and strokes. They will also look and feel better. In addition to the use of diet and supplements a variety of other complementary therapies are of great benefit in improving fertility.

Marilyn has an international reputation for researching her subject meticulously and comprehensively and then distilling the essential components. This book is an excellent example of how complex theory may successfully be put into simple practice. The subjects are explained clearly and sympathetically with a wealth of practical tips and advice. The book takes the reader by the hand and guides them along the path to successful conception.

Marilyn has a warm, down-to-earth and supportive approach that shines through every page. This combination of professional expertise and excellence and deep humanity makes this book a gem. I would recommend this book to couples having difficulty conceiving as well as couples thinking of starting a family.

Yehudi Gordon MB, Bch, MD, FRCOG
Consultant gynaecologist and obstetrician
December 1999

Acknowledgements

There are a number of people I would like to thank for their help and support with this book.

I would especially like to thank Maggie Drummond for her help in making this book so readable. Special thanks also go to Rachel Winning, my editor at Piatkus, for her invaluable input and to the staff of Piatkus for their expertise.

As always, the staff at my practice have enabled me to take the time to write this book and have kept the practice running as smoothly as ever. I would particularly like to thank, Linda McVan, my practice manager, and also Bea, Lou, Trish, Susie and Sue.

My love goes to my husband Kriss and my children Matthew, Leonard and Chantell for their love and encouragement.

Sincere admiration goes to Belinda Barnes the Founder of Foresight. For over 20 years she has championed the need for preconception care and has achieved so much in that time with respect to the awareness that the months before conception are as vital as the pregnancy itself. At the beginning she was a lone voice, but over time this has changed especially with the scientific research confirming what she already knew.

My deepest respect and appreciation goes to the team at Reproductive Health Care for their commitment to the highest possible standards of fertility investigations, treatment and total emotional and physical care of the couples who come to the clinic. I would especially like to thank Yehudi Gordon, consultant gynaecologist, for his open-mindedness and willingness to incorporate Integrated Medicine (the coming together of conventional and complementary medicine) into his clinic. Yehudi has always been a pioneer, first in the area of natural birth and now in other areas of women's health. Integrated Medicine will be the medicine of the future, and is of particular interest to Prince Charles who instigated the setting up of the Foundation for Integrated Medicine, but it is another thing to see it happening in practice.

My special thanks also go to Talha Shwaf, consultant gynaecologist and reproductive medicine specialist for his invaluable expertise and discussions regarding the technical aspects of this book. I am very grateful to him for reading through the draft and for his constructive criticisms.

'Today's unorthodoxy is probably going to be tomorrow's convention'
HRH The Prince of Wales, BMA President 1982–3

Introduction

Over the last two decades, there has been a significant rise in the number of couples experiencing fertility problems:

- Sperm counts have dropped by 50 per cent in the last ten years.[1]
- Men are showing an increasing number of sperm abnormalities.
- A quarter of all couples planning a baby have trouble conceiving.
- It is not uncommon for a couple without any fertility problems to take two to three years to conceive.
- One in four women miscarry. Some experience repeated miscarriages – as often as ten times.
- More and more couples are turning to fertility treatments to enable them to have a family.
- Of the couples who seek medical help, 30 per cent are told they have 'unexplained infertility' for which the doctors can offer no treatment.

If you are reading this book, you or your partner may have experienced problems trying to have a baby. You may have gone through fertility treatments that failed. Or you may just be worried that nothing is happening. I see hundreds of couples every year who are trying to conceive and I fully understand their unhappiness and frustration at not being able to achieve something that most of us grew up believing would happen whenever we wanted.

But, as the above statistics reveal, you are not alone. There is an epidemic of infertility and subfertility – and in many cases the doctors do not know the answers.

But, before we discuss these issues, I want to say:

Don't lose heart

I believe that getting yourself and your partner into optimum health, using the four-month programme outlined in this book, will give you the best possible chance of having that longed-for, healthy baby.

I don't just believe it – I *know* it. By the time you have finished reading this book, I hope I will have inspired you and your partner to take control of your health and fertility.

Nature is wonderfully clever. At this particular moment you may not think so, because on the most fundamental level, reproduction, it seems to have let you down. But the purpose of this book is to encourage you to restore your own and your partner's fertility to its proper 'natural' state by simple lifestyle and dietary changes that eliminate toxins from your body and ensure that you have the level of nutrients needed for conception.

Fundamentals of Health

In the animal world, fertility is paramount for the survival of any species. However, the human race today has a number of fertility problems. Men are showing sperm abnormalities (such as sperm with two heads or sperm that are so sluggish they cannot reach the egg). Some women have a number of menstrual cycles during which they do not ovulate; or, when fertilisation happens, the embryo does not implant in the womb.

To explain these anomalies, we have to go back to the foundations of health. The egg and sperm are only as healthy as the man and woman who produce them. If there are any problems with either the egg or the sperm, however subtle, nature will either try to stop fertilisation occurring or, if it does take place, a miscarriage may follow.

One reason why so many couples are diagnosed with 'unexplained infertility' is that doctors cannot put it down to a specific, observable medical cause. But I believe that infertility is a multi-factorial problem and should be investigated that way. That means looking at a variety of issues, such as nutrition, alcohol and smoking habits, levels of lead and other toxic metals, pesticides, food additives, genito-urinary infections, allergies, stress and other hazards of modern life. That means your partner taking a close look at *his* health and nutrition as well (in four out of ten cases of infertility, the problems are on the male side). The fact is that our modern 'unnatural' lifestyle, combined with the nutrient depletion of much of our food, has left many of us deficient in the vitamins and minerals we need for successful babymaking.

Any specialist who works in a zoo, or breeds champion dogs, cattle or racehorses, will tell you that optimum nutrition is essential. But, while the fertility clinic business is booming (with desperate couples lining up for treatment), there isn't much incentive to look at whether simple factors, like a deficiency of zinc for instance, may be the main reason for unexplained infertility.

Learning From the Past

We should learn from the folic acid story, which really demonstrates the importance of nutrition and how a crucial deficiency identified by researchers as being responsible for birth abnormalities was ignored by doctors for years.

In 1991 the Medical Research Council (MRC) finally published a study which showed that supplementing with folic acid during preconception and pregnancy could prevent the reccurrence of spina bifida in babies.[2] Yet the damaging effects of a folic acid deficiency had been recognised three decades earlier, after rats were born with malformations (including neural tube defects) and other problems (such as club foot and cleft palate) in folic acid trials.[3]

This knowledge, which could have prevented a great deal of heartache, had been around for over 30 years and yet women were not told to take folic acid for decades. These early findings were confirmed again in humans in 1981 trials that looked at the effects of folic acid on the prevention of spina bifida.[4]

Even as recently as 1993 the *Daily Mail* ran an article asking 'Could this vitamin save your baby?'[5] It said, 'The fact that a supplement which can stop women having spina bifida babies remains the best kept secret of preconceptual care has now prompted sharp criticism from the medical world.'

Cynically, one might suppose that if folic acid had not been a simple easy-to-obtain supplement but a highly profitable pharmaceutical drug we would all have known about it years ago. You cannot patent a nutrient so there is no commercial incentive to investigate and promote it.

But the big lesson we should learn from the folic acid story is that our diet – what we eat or don't eat – is absolutely crucial to our fertility.

How to Use This Book

Folic acid is only the tip of the iceberg. Medical and scientific literature contains a great deal of information that can help couples who are having difficulty conceiving or who have had previous problems such as miscarriages and malformations. This book presents that information in an easy-to-understand form so that you can use it yourself. Having this knowledge will help you gain control of your own health and fertility.

By following the advice in this book you can increase your fertility and reduce the possibility of miscarriage. Even if you have a condition like blocked fallopian tubes (which means that you need IVF treatment in order to have a chance of conceiving), this book will increase your chance of success. With assisted conception techniques it is still vital for the sperm and the egg to be as healthy as possible.

As you read the recommendations, you'll realise that the changes you make to increase your fertility are the same as those that will protect you from miscarriage and help you produce a healthy baby. They are also, quite simply, recommendations that will improve your general health. The advice is so logical and makes such sense that you will probably wonder why no one has told you all this before.

Finding that you can't conceive when you want is a real shock and it is not something that many of us want to talk about even to our close friends and families. GPs and consultants are busy people and, all too often, overworked. The minute you come out of the consulting room you think of a dozen other things you wanted to discuss. There just isn't time to talk in as much depth as you would like. Yet you want to find out as much as you can. This book is designed to answer your specific queries as well as present a comprehensive self-help programme that will give you and your partner the best chance of conceiving.

- **Section 1** outlines the different aspects of your life and health that could be causing your and your partner's problem. This will help you identify what may be going wrong.

- **Section 2** explains how you can help improve your and your partner's fertility, concentrating particularly on good nutrition and supplementing your diet. This is one of the most crucial sections in the book because it could be the key to solving your infertility problem by making some simple changes that are entirely within your own control.

- **Section 3** explains what tests are available to help you identify any medical cause of infertility. It is important that your partner understands that he must also be involved in this process.

- **Section 4** describes the different fertility treatments available in the UK and reveals some heartening evidence that you and your partner can dramatically improve your chances of having successful fertility treatment, if you should need it, by following the advice in this book.

- **Section 5** discusses the problem of miscarriage in depth and shows how you can help yourself overcome it.

- **Section 6** puts it all into practice – and shows you how to organise your self-help programme for those vital months of preparation. This is really the most essential part of the book.

- **Section 7** tells you how to care for yourself in pregnancy so as to ensure that you will have a healthy baby.

I believe that any couple planning to have a baby would benefit from following the kind of recommendations outlined in this book – not just couples who have had problems conceiving.

If all this sounds too hard to stick to, just think how important it is . . . We plan our holidays and we train for a career so why should we expect to just have babies without any proper planning or preparation? This preconception care period of three or four months shapes your baby's future, both physically and mentally, so it could be the most important bit of planning you ever do in your life. My aim is to help you and your partner to optimum health to give you both the best chance of having a healthy baby. As a bonus, following these recommendations will make you both feel better, fitter and more energetic.

Self-help Strategies

Most couples who seek fertility treatment find out a great deal about sophisticated medical technologies but very little about the relatively simple measures they themselves can take to improve their chances of conceiving. These highly effective self-help strategies include easily implemented dietary and lifestyle changes. Such measures cost little or nothing, their success has been scientifically documented, and yet most of these couples will not have been told about them. Why on earth is this?

The cynical answer is that infertility has become 'big business'. As Professor Robert Winston points out in his book *Making Babies*, there are now at least 21 IVF units in London alone. And more and more units are opening because they are 'highly profitable in the private sector'. Couples who desperately want to have a baby are very vulnerable. Even though some IVF units have extremely low success rates, such couples are still willing to gamble a great deal of time and money in order to try to conceive.

In contrast, there are no big financial gains to be made in helping couples to look at their lifestyle or to correct their vitamin and mineral deficiencies. Yet this approach makes such sense, and has been shown to give an unprecedented success rate.

Over the last 20 years, Foresight has pioneered an approach to fertility that looks at the fundamentals of health, including lifestyle, diet, pollutants, infections and environmental and occupational hazards and gives an unprecedented 80 per cent success rate. Researchers from the University of Surrey followed the progress of 367 couples over a period of three years (1990–3). The women were aged between 22 and 45, and the men were aged 25 to 59. In all, 37 per cent of the couples had a history of infertility, and 38 per cent had experienced between one and five miscarriages (others had had other problems, including still births, malformations and low birth-weight babies).

Many of the couples were older, coming to the trial as a 'last resort'. They were all asked to eliminate smoking and alcohol, and to follow the recommendations outlined in this book (such as buying organic food, having infections checked and having mineral analysis). All the couples were given personal supplement programmes and were then re-tested to make sure their levels had returned to normal.

By the end of the three-year trial, 89 per cent (327 of the couples) had given birth. Out of those couples with a previous history of infertility, 81 per cent conceived and had babies. Out of those who had experienced a previous miscarriage, 83 per cent had a baby within the three years of the study, without experiencing another miscarriage.

Of the 327 babies born to the couples in the study, no baby was born before 36 weeks and none was lighter than 5lb 2oz (2.368kg). There were no miscarriages, perinatal deaths or malformations. The national average for miscarriages is one in four so one could at least have expected 80 miscarriages, but there were none. No baby was admitted to a special care baby unit.

A number of the couples had already tried IVF – sometimes two or three times – without success. Yet 65 per cent of this group conceived naturally on the Foresight programme without needing another IVF cycle.

These results are undeniably impressive and speak for themselves. Yet sceptics maintain that they are 'too good to be true'. To date, the results have been published in the *Journal of Nutritional and Environmental Medicine* but not in a standard medical journal.[6] This is because, in order to be accepted by a medical journal, there must be a control group.

In a normal double-blind placebo controlled trial, to assess the efficacy of a headache remedy, for example, volunteers are randomly assigned to either a control group (placebo) or a treatment group (headache remedy). The volunteers don't know if they are taking the placebo or the remedy, and nor does the scientist running the trial. All the volunteers in the treated group get the same dose of headache remedy.

However, in this study each person was given an individual supplement programme according to their needs. So they were all taking different dosages and supplements, depending on how deficient or toxic they were.

This is an important point because the double-blind placebo controlled trial is the 'gold standard' in medicine but it cannot take into account that we are all unique and that we may need different treatments to increase our fertility. And it is this 'individually tailored' approach which I believe is the key to finding a natural solution to infertility. The fact is that 37 per cent of the couples in this study had an established history of fertility problems and had undergone medical investigation. They did something different – changed their dietary habits and lifestyle – and then conceived. The information contained in this book explains in detail my enhanced version of this pre-conception programme.

It worked for them. It could work for you.

FACTORS THAT CAN AFFECT YOUR FERTILITY

Conception is a complex process that depends on everything working properly at a number of stages.

Firstly, your hormone balance must be correct so that the egg develops normally. Secondly, you must be ovulating so that the egg is released. Thirdly, you must have sex at the right time in your cycle (there may be only two or three days a month when you are fertile). In addition, your partner must have a good sperm count and possess healthy sperm, which are capable of penetrating your cervical mucus to reach the egg. Then the egg has to be captured by the fallopian tube and be fertilised. Finally, once the egg has been fertilised, the embryo has to implant securely in the lining of the womb, which needs the right levels of the hormone progesterone to maintain the pregnancy. No wonder they talk about the miracle of life!

It's daunting to think about the number of things that can go wrong. But, as we have seen, there are many simple ways in which you can dramatically improve your chances of getting pregnant.

In this section of the book I outline all the different factors that can undermine your fertility. The list may seem long but it is important to identify the particular combination of factors that may be undermining your and your partner's health and wellbeing.

You may have been given the impression that there is no medical reason – and therefore no solution – for your problem. But when you read this section you will realise that nothing could be further from the truth.

CHAPTER 1

Nutrition

You are what you eat. Or, to put it another way, if you put poor-quality petrol in a high-performance car, like a Rolls-Royce or a Porsche, it may run for a while but eventually it will become less productive and less efficient. It is exactly the same with the human body. You need top-grade 'fuel' to function properly, and to produce healthy eggs or sperm. To a very large extent, your fertility depends on what you eat.

Food Isn't What it Used to Be

One of the problems is that nowadays we eat a lot of convenience and refined foods that have been stripped of essential nutrients during manufacturing. For example, 80 per cent of zinc is removed from wheat during the milling process to ensure that a loaf of bread has a longer shelf life.[7]

The soil our food is grown on is so lacking in nutrients due to overuse and commercial farming methods, that even what we regard as 'healthy' foods – vegetables, for instance – may not contain the amounts of minerals we expect to get from them. If you have been dieting for a number of years (either restricting your food intake or trying different diet drinks or pills), you could well be deficient in a number of vitamins and minerals.

The well-balanced diet is a myth. We simply do not get all the nutrients we need from our food. This was confirmed by a National Food Survey conducted in 1995 which found that the average person in Britain was grossly deficient in six out of the eight vitamins and minerals surveyed. Fewer than one in ten people received the RDA (Recommended Daily Allowance) for zinc, which is the most important mineral for both male and female fertility.

Put this lack of nutrients together with all the additives, preservatives and pesticides (see Chapters 4 and 5) in your food and you can see that your fertility may well be compromised on a daily basis. Chemicals like pesticides are known to affect fertility, others will affect your general health, and this in turn can reduce your ability to conceive. Scientists may know the toxic effects of one particular chemical but what they don't and can't know for certain is the effect of being exposed to a cocktail of these substances.

Balancing the Scales

Your weight is crucial for your fertility. Being very underweight or very overweight can make conception difficult or impossible. So it's important that your weight is within a certain range in order to give you the best chance of conceiving.

Nature gave women proportionately more body fat for a specific purpose, in order to reproduce and then feed our young. That is why fat accounts for 27 per cent of an average woman's body weight, while it is only 15 per cent for a man.

Fat is essential to fertility and it is necessary in order to ovulate. Young girls do not begin to menstruate until their bodies are composed of at least 17 per cent fat.

Underweight

If a woman's body fat drops too low, then her periods can stop. This low level of body fat may be caused by excessive exercise, as sometimes happens with ballet dancers or athletes who have very tough physical regimes.[8]

Infertility can also be caused by excessive dieting. When a woman is anorexic, for instance, her periods stop.[9] With so much publicity about anorexia and an increasing number of young women falling victim to the 'slimmer's disease', the long-term damage to fertility caused by drastic weight loss is well-known. But not so many people realise that being overweight can also affect fertility.

Overweight

If a woman is overweight it can stop her ovulating. Studies have shown that just losing a small amount of weight, 10 per cent, for instance, can be enough to increase fertility by stimulating ovulation, improving hormone balance and making periods more regular.[10]

In another study, on women who previously did not ovulate, 11 out of 12 conceived naturally after exercising and dieting over a period of six months to get their weight down.[11]

Fortunately your dietary intake is fully within your control, and eating the right food may be the single most important thing you can do to achieve a successful pregnancy. Later (in Chapter 7) I will explain how the right nutrition can give you and your partner optimum health and fertility.

CHAPTER 2

Alcohol, Smoking and Drugs

Most of us know that smoking and drinking alcohol when pregnant can be very harmful to the baby. But what most couples don't realise is that smoking and alcohol could actually be stopping them conceiving a baby because it reduces their fertility. The good news is that the negative effects are not permanent and simply stopping will dramatically improve your chances.

Alcohol

Research has shown that drinking alcohol causes a decrease in sperm count, an increase in abnormal sperm and a lower proportion of motile sperm.[12]

Alcohol also affects a man's fertility by changing his hormone levels because it can alter the way testosterone is produced and then released.[13] Because alcohol affects the liver (the organ which normally clears out any excess hormones), a man who drinks alcohol may accumulate small amounts of female hormones (men produce 'female' hormones, just as women produce testosterone). These female hormones can lower sperm production and potency.

In addition, alcohol stops absorption of nutrients like zinc which is one of the most important minerals for male fertility. Zinc is found in high concentrations in the sperm. Adequate levels of zinc are needed to make the outer layer and tail and are therefore essential for healthy sperm. If you reduce the amount of zinc in a man's diet, his sperm count goes down.[14]

Finally, alcohol reduces fertility in mammals, and studies show that women who drink heavily may stop ovulating and menstruating, and take longer to conceive.[15]

How Much is Too Much?

A study of 430 women demonstrated that drinking more than 5 units of alcohol (equal to five glasses of wine) a week could stop women conceiving. Researchers discovered that the women in the survey who drank less than 5 units a week were twice as likely to get pregnant within six months compared with those who drank more. A study published in the *British Medical Journal* concluded that women should be 'warned to avoid alcohol when trying to conceive'.[16]

The fact is that drinking *any* alcohol can reduce your fertility by half – and the more you drink, the worse the impact on your chances of conception.[17]

Studies have also shown a strong relationship between alcohol and miscarriages. Women who have a drink every day have a much higher risk of miscarriage (2.5 times more) than non-drinkers.[18] The same study found that if the woman was a drinker and a smoker her chance of a miscarriage was four times higher.

Smoking

There is so much information available nowadays about the risks of lung cancer, emphysema and other life-threatening conditions and most people are aware of the detrimental effects of smoking when pregnant. I know how shocked many of us feel when we see a heavily pregnant woman standing with a cigarette in her hand. Yet most people are not aware of the impact smoking can have on a couple's fertility. It's not surprising that tobacco has such an effect – it contains more than 4,000 compounds, including carbon monoxide, oxide of nitrogen, ammonia, aromatic hydrocarbons, hydrogen cyanide, vinylchloride, nicotine, lead and cadmium.

Although many women smokers resolve to give up when they get pregnant, they don't realise that by smoking they are reducing their chances of getting pregnant in the first place. Not only that but you don't usually know that you are pregnant for the first couple of weeks and the baby will be taking in all that tobacco smoke in the meantime.

The man's fertility is also affected by smoking – it decreases his sperm count, makes his sperm more sluggish, increases the number of abnormal sperm and reduces his testosterone levels.

In addition, smoking reduces the level of vitamin C in the bloodstream. Lack of vitamin C encourages sperm to clump together (a process known as agglutination) instead of moving forward to fertilise the egg. One study showed how male fertility was improved by giving men 500mg of vitamin C twice a day.[19]

Smoking has definitely been linked with infertility in women.[20] It can even bring on an early menopause, which is an especially important consideration for older women trying to conceive who may be racing against time.[21] If you are a smoker, you should ask yourself why you are taking something into your body that is bringing you nearer to the menopause – and infertility?

Recreational Drugs

The use of marijuana and cocaine has increased steadily over the years to the point where, for some people, it is part of everyday life. Although still illegal, recreational drug use is increasingly socially acceptable. That does not mean it is healthy or safe. The fact is that these drugs can compromise both your and your partner's fertility. But, as with alcohol and tobacco, you can stop using recreational drugs and negate the damage to your fertility in a relatively short space of time.

If you continue to use them during a pregnancy, of course, it can have disastrous effects on your developing baby.

The Effects of Some Common Recreational Drugs

- **Marijuana** can lower a man's levels of FSH and LH, two hormones needed to produce sperm. It can also lower his libido.[22] For the woman, marijuana can lead to irregular periods, reducing fertility and sometimes even stopping ovulation.[23]

- **Cocaine** users will have a lower sperm count, poorly moving sperm and a high rate of abnormal sperm.[24]

- **Heroin** can cause a decrease in testosterone levels.[25]

- **Cocaine and heroin**, taken together, will make it harder for a woman to conceive and she is more likely to have a miscarriage, a stillbirth or a baby born with a malformation.[26]

Medicines

If you or your partner are taking medication while you are trying to conceive you should speak to your doctor about which drugs are medically essential and which are not. Some drugs have a direct effect on fertility and you do need to discuss this with your GP.

Many drugs can affect not only the man's sperm but also his ejaculatory function and libido. Some medicines may even cause impotence. These drugs can include sulphasalazine (used to treat irritable bowel), nitrofurantoin, tetracyclines, cimetidine, ketoconazole, tricyclic antidepressants, monoamine oxidase inhibitors and propranol.[27]

In addition, medication given for conditions like gout or high blood pressure can interfere with fertility. And non-steroidal anti-inflammatory drugs (often used for arthritis) can stop ovulation.[28]

CHAPTER 3

Age and Medical Problems

Age

The bad news is that the older we get, the less fertile we become – and that goes for men as well as women. A woman's eggs have been in her body since before she was born, so that means that at the age of 35 those eggs are older than they were when she was 25. This is one reason why fertility declines after the age of 35. It can take longer to get pregnant and the risk of miscarriage is higher. Biologically, it is more efficient for women to have their families when they are young. But, in recent years, the average age of women having their first baby has been going up because many of us now want to establish ourselves in a career before starting families.

Women going through fertility investigations are often told that they are not conceiving because they have 'old eggs'. The use of this term has a devastating psychological effect on any woman. And it causes a lot of unnecessary heartache because, although you cannot increase the number of eggs you have left, it is very possible to improve their quality by improving your general health.

So, if you are over the age of 35, rest assured that there is a great deal you can do to increase your fertility – and these strategies are discussed in detail in Section 2. You can also take heart from the story of Sarah, a 42-year-old, who came to me for advice.

Case History

Sarah, a solicitor, was absolutely distraught after her third attempt at IVF treatment. She had been told that the quality of her eggs was no good and

---

that she was now menopausal. She had not responded well to her last course of IVF drugs. But when she asked whether the drugs could perhaps be altered she was told that there was nothing wrong with the technology; she was the problem. You can imagine how devastated she felt. She had emerged from the clinic with the words 'old eggs' ringing in her ears.

I told her there was no guarantee but I would aim to get her and her partner in optimum health, which would be of benefit anyway. They followed the plan outlined in Section 6 of this book (taking supplements, and making changes to their diet and lifestyle).

Six months later Sarah was pregnant, and she has since had a healthy baby boy.

Medical Problems

There are a number of medical conditions that can affect fertility. Some are directly linked to the reproductive process, such as blocked fallopian tubes. Some, like coeliac disease, are not obviously linked. However, many of these conditions can be treated (see Section 3). And, by improving your general health and fitness, you can do a great deal to help overcome these problems and regain your fertility.

Conditions Affecting Female Fertility

Blocked Fallopian Tubes

The fallopian tubes are the route between the ovaries and the womb. The sperm swim along these tubes in order to reach the egg. The fallopian tube also provides a home for the fertilised egg for the first seven days of life, before it gets to the womb where it will implant itself. If the tubes are blocked then this is a major problem and medical intervention is needed.

Polycystic Ovary Syndrome

Polycystic ovary syndrome (PCOS) is the main reason why some women stop ovulating.[29] In its most extreme form, it can be a very distressing condition. Women affected by PCOS will tend to be overweight, prone to acne, menstruate seldom or not at all, grow unsightly body hair (often on the face, breasts and inside of the legs), and be susceptible to mood swings.

Fibroids

Fibroids are non-cancerous growths which grow in or on the wall of the womb. They are very common and many women never realise they have them, as they may not cause any symptoms. If they grow in a way that doesn't exert pressure on neighbouring organs, a woman can live with large fibroids for many years without needing medical help. They can, however, cause infertility and some fibroids can cause miscarriages (see Section 5). Fibroids can vary in number and size. If the fibroids grow significantly they can cause the uterus to enlarge and/or distort which makes it difficult for the embryo to implant properly. So you might conceive easily but miscarry unawares, at a very early stage, because the fertilised egg could not 'hold on' with the fibroid there. The size of a fibroid is usually compared to a foetus of that size (e.g. a 12-week fibroid) but some can be as small as a pea.

Endometriosis

Endometriosis is a condition where the lining of the womb (the endometrium) grows in places other than the womb. Sections of womb lining may grow in the fallopian tubes, ovaries, bowel and bladder. More uncommon places include the lung, heart, eye or knee. The womb lining, no matter where it is situated, then responds to the natural hormone cycle and will bleed when the period occurs. This can be extremely painful, especially in those sites where there is no natural escape route for the blood, and inflammation may occur. For instance, I have seen women who get a nose bleed during their period because the womb lining has migrated to the nasal passages and bleeds when they menstruate.

Endometriosis can affect female fertility because it can cause scarring and blockages inside the pelvic cavity, and it is thought that 50 per cent of women with endometriosis may have problems getting pregnant. It is more common in women over 30 who have not had children. So, as more women delay having children, the possibility of infertility being caused by endometriosis rises.

In some cases the endometriosis scars and obstructs the fallopian tubes so severely that the tubes cannot pick up the egg. And if the ovaries are scarred badly then ovulation may not occur. When the endometrial tissue implants on the ovary then cysts may form called 'chocolate cysts' because they are filled with dark, brown, old blood.

Coeliac Disease

This is a medical condition caused by an intolerance to gluten which prevents food being absorbed properly. Symptoms can include foul-smelling greasy stools, weight loss, anaemia, bloating, fatigue, and signs of multiple vitamin and mineral deficiencies.

Unfortunately, coeliac disease can also cause fertility problems. A study in 1996 confirmed that women with coeliac disease were subfertile and had an increased risk of stillbirths and perinatal deaths.[30]

Gluten is a major component of wheat; and other cereals, such as rye, barley and oats, can also be a problem. Rice and corn are fine. The gluten damages the villi, which are minute, hair-like projections lining the intestine, and this can stop the absorption of vital nutrients. The disorder is diagnosed by having a biopsy in which a sample of the small intestine is removed for examination.

Conditions Affecting Male Fertility

Up to 40 per cent of couples' infertility problems can turn out to be on the man's side but the focus is still, generally, on the woman. From the beginning your partner should be involved in finding out what is preventing both of you from getting pregnant and tackling the problem – it could well be a combination of factors.

Here are some common conditions that make men less fertile. Many of them can be helped by making the simple changes described in Section 2, and most of them can be investigated using the tests described in Chapter 16.

Low Sperm Count

If his sperm count is low (less than 20 million per millilitre) then this could definitely be reducing your chances of conceiving. Levels of 40 million would be much better.

Poor Sperm Movement

Even if there is a good sperm count, fertility will be affected if the sperm's capacity to move itself along (its 'motility') is poor. The way the sperm move is important because if they are going round and round in circles they won't be able to travel up through the cervix and into the uterus to reach the egg. Good motility is also needed to help the sperm penetrate the egg.

Agglutination

This is when sperm clump together in a circle, going nowhere. This can be caused by an infection or by antibodies (see page 141).

Abnormal Sperm

All men have a percentage of abnormal sperm and up to 70 per cent is considered acceptable. The abnormal sperm can have two heads or no tails, for example. But only if there is a very high percentage of abnormal sperm will a man's fertility be affected.

Many specialists believe that these abnormal sperm would find it difficult to get to the fallopian tube and, once there, would not be able to penetrate an egg. But some studies have shown that abnormal sperm are actually capable of reaching the fallopian tube.[31]

Others claim that a high concentration of abnormal sperm could be connected with a high rate of miscarriages.[32]

Research has shown that, while the possibility of conception increases with higher sperm counts, it is also vital that the sperm are normal. One study, published in the *Lancet* in 1998, showed that a man with a lower sperm count can still be fertile as long as there is a high proportion of normal sperm.[33]

Varicoceles

These are enlarged veins around the testes. They need not cause any discomfort and do not affect the man's health in any way. However, it is thought that they can overheat the testes and damage sperm production, though there are men who have varicoceles and do not have any fertility problems. For some men with infertility, tying off these veins has helped them conceive. For other men, it has made no difference at all. Unfortunately doctors cannot predict which men with varicoceles will benefit from having them treated.

Obstructions

Blockages in certain parts of the male reproductive system can affect fertility by stopping sperm getting through to be ejaculated. These blockages can occur because of scarring caused by an infection such as mycoplasma or ureaplasma (see page 23), or because of previous surgery, or due to an injury (e.g. a kick in the groin while playing sport). A severe sports injury could also stop the testes producing sperm.

Undescended Testes

If the testes did not come down properly after birth, then they may not be producing sperm. The incidence of this problem is increasing and many scientists now feel that (like the drop in sperm count) it is related to environmental factors. (The impact of these environmental factors is discussed in Chapter 4.) Surgery is often used to bring down a young boy's testes (which, earlier in childhood, have got stuck inside the body) into the scrotum. If undescended testes were not diagnosed early enough and surgery was delayed then the man's fertility may have been affected.

Diseases

Glandular diseases, such as thyroid or diabetes mellitus, can interfere with hormonal control of sperm production. Infections of the prostate and epididymis (tubular structure on top of each of the testes, into which secretions drain) can interfere with sperm production or block the exit of sperm from the body. Other infections such as mumps orchitis (an inflammation of the testicles following the mumps) can result in permanent infertility.

Infections Affecting Both Male and Female Fertility

Many people don't realise there are a number of infections that can damage fertility. Some can cause infertility in both men and women, some can stop the embryo implanting once fertilisation has taken place, and some can cause miscarriages.

In men, infections in the seminal vesicles or the prostate gland can affect the sperm in several ways. Pus cells will reduce the sperm's swimming ability and certain infections may kill off the sperm. Some infections can cause blockages in the male reproductive system, stopping the effective transport of the sperm. Cytomegalovirus (CMV), which is caused by a herpes virus, has been linked with low sperm count and inflammation of the testes.[34]

Chlamydia

Chlamydia may sound like an exotic flower but it is actually a sexually transmitted bacteria which can lead to infertility in women without causing any symptoms. It is effectively an infertility timebomb, which is claiming growing numbers of victims (particularly teenage girls). The Royal College of Physicians' Committee on Genito-urinary Medicine estimates that it is the most common sexually transmitted disease in our society.[35]

A number of countries, such as Sweden, routinely screen for chlamydia trachomatis and the fall in the number of chlamydia cases there has been dramatic. But there is no routine screening in the UK. It is known as the 'silent illness' because only a small number of women experience actual symptoms such as a discharge. Men can also get chlamydia. They feel a burning sensation on passing urine. If men do not get the symptoms investigated then they will infect their partners, and possibly damage their own fertility.

In a woman the chlamydia bacteria can lie dormant for many months before passing through the cervix, and from there unnoticed into the womb and up the fallopian tubes where it causes the majority of pelvic inflammatory diseases (PID). If untreated, it can damage the fallopian tubes, resulting in blocked or scarred tubes which can mean infertility or increased risk of an ectopic pregnancy (where the fertilised egg implants into the fallopian tube instead of in the womb). In men it can cause inflammation of the testes and the tubes surrounding the testes.[36]

Women can be screened for chlamydia with a cervical swab and/or a urine test and men can have a urine test. If caught early it can be treated successfully with antibiotics.

Mycoplasma and Ureaplasma

Mycoplasma hominis and *Ureaplasma urealyticum* are very common organisms that can infect the genito-urinary tracts of men and women. These organisms don't always cause infertility, *but*:

- According to a study in the 1970s, there seems to be a higher frequency of these organisms in the ejaculates and cervical secretions of couples with unexplained infertility problems. And when the couples were treated, pregnancy rates increased.[39]

• In men, this type of infection can decrease the sperm count, reduce motility and increase the number of abnormal sperm.[40]

• These organisms have also been linked with an increased risk of miscarriage.[41]

CHAPTER 4

Environmental Hazards

We live in a society where we are bombarded with chemicals and toxins. All the time we are exposed to chemicals in our food, in the packaging around it, in pesticides, additives and preservatives. In our houses, we can be in contact with chemicals through household cleaners, aerosols, new carpets treated with moth-proofing, and anti-woodworm and wood preservation treatments.

Outside, the environment is equally laden with toxins – traffic fumes, factory pollution, pesticides sprayed on parks and railways. Dangerous chemicals seep out from landfill sites. The list goes on . . .

All this affects your fertility. Logic tells us that toxins must be one of the main reasons why an increasing number of couples face difficulties conceiving. The fact is that we are living in a 'sea' of hormones.

Of course it's difficult to link a specific chemical to a particular medical problem or illness. So much else in our lives may affect our health that it's often impossible to isolate the real culprits.

But we can learn a lot from the animal world. Infertility in wildlife is known to be linked to substances called xenoestrogens, oestrogen-like chemicals in the environment caused by pollution from pesticides and the manufacturing of plastics.

The power of these xenoestrogens was demonstrated when a group of scientists discovered that alligators which had hatched in Lake Apopka, Florida, had abnormally small penises and altered hormonal levels. In 1980 there had been a massive spill of Kelthane pesticide into the lake – the xenoestrogens from the pesticide were feminising the alligators and stopping reproduction.

Meanwhile, in the UK, the Department for the Environment found hermaphrodite fish in one river. The fish were part male and part female.

In view of all this it seems very likely that chemicals in regular use are having a damaging impact on our fertility.

Genetically Modified Foods

Fortunately the issue of genetically modified foods has provoked a groundswell of opposition amongst the British public. We were just recovering from the BSE crisis when suddenly our food faced another threat. If the commercial production of GM foods goes ahead in Britain, we could find ourselves sitting on yet another health timebomb – possibly the most devastating of all.

GM foods are already affecting the fertility of insects that feed on them. For example, ladybirds that ate greenfly fed on genetically modified potatoes had a drastic reduction in fertility, with fewer eggs being produced.

Likewise, when a gene to produce redness was put into a petunia, it produced plants with more roots, hairier leaves and a reduction in fertility. Scientists should know by now that they cannot manipulate nature without consequences.

Household Chemicals

Think about the number of chemicals we have in our houses – all those cleaners and aerosols. There is plenty of evidence that the chemicals they contain can be harmful.

In an American study, published in 1991, women with a history of unexplained infertility and recurrent miscarriages were found to have high levels of two chemicals commonly found in carpets, leather upholstery and wood preservatives.[42]

Leading UK fertility expert Lord Professor Robert Winston believes that chemicals in emulsion paint being used in a closed laboratory over 100 metres away from his clinic affected embryo growth at a vital stage of treatment. No one is allowed to wear perfume or aftershave in Lord Winston's clinic because he believes it is important to avoid chemicals when trying to maximise fertility. Some chemicals can stop women conceiving, or the egg may fertilise naturally but not be able to grow or develop.

Ionising Radiation

This type of radiation – which gives off charged particles called ions – is produced from X-rays. It has the power to change cells and can cause infertility and miscarriages.

The male testis is one of the most radio-sensitive tissues and must be carefully protected during routine X-rays. Studies have shown that even low doses of X-ray delivered directly to the testes can reduce the sperm count temporarily to zero.[43] If the same dose is split up over time, instead of being given in one go, recovery of the sperm can take up to ten years.[44] Clearly, men exposed to X-rays through their work are likely to have reduced sperm counts.[45]

Non-ionising Radiation

This does not create ions and is produced naturally by the sun. We are exposed to it every day through microwaves, radar, mobile phones, radio waves, televisions, computers, electric blankets, etc.

Mobile Phones

There have been lots of scary stories in the media about the dangers of mobile phones. It has been claimed that they can cause a harmful rise in blood pressure. Other research has found that regular users have more headaches. And there are concerns that mobile phones can cause 'hot spots' in the brain, with a possible link to brain tumours. But investigators have stressed that more research needs to be done.

Meanwhile, scientists at the University of Montpellier in France have found that chick embryos can be damaged by electromagnetic signals sent out by VDUs and televisions.[46] When chick embryos were exposed to mobile phone radiation during the 21-day incubation period there was a five-fold increase in chick deaths, which suggests that there might be an increased risk of miscarriage in humans. The possible increased risk of miscarriage and the effects on human male and female fertility have not yet been investigated.

Microwave Cooking

The first microwaves went on sale in the UK in 1974 and now almost three-quarters of British households own a microwave oven. A microwave oven heats food by using high-frequency electromagnetic waves, similar to television. The molecules of the food agitate at over 2,000 times per second so that the food heats itself. The idea is that the metal oven is a sealed unit: microwaves cannot penetrate metal so they cannot escape. However, most of the health concerns have centred on the possibility that radiation could be leaking out during cooking and affecting fertility. There are also worries that food cooked in a microwave may be inherently changed in ways we are not yet aware of.

Because microwaving does not use water, vitamins which are water-soluble (like vitamin C) are conserved in the food. For example, potatoes keep 82 per cent of their vitamin C when they are microwaved, as compared to 40 per cent when they are boiled.

But microwaving tends to destroy the fat-soluble vitamins, like vitamins A, D and E. Pumpkin seeds, which have valuable amounts of essential fatty acids, lose 46 per cent of these oils after 10 minutes of irradiation.[47] These essential fatty acids, as you will see in Section 2, are vital for both male and female fertility.

Microwave cooking also seems to destroy the cell walls of plant foods like vegetables. Studies on microwaved carrots and broccoli show that the molecular structure is deformed, whereas in conventional cooking the cell structure stays intact.[48]

What this means is that the microwave process seems to encourage the production of free radicals (highly reactive chemical fragments which have been linked to cancer, coronary heart disease, rheumatoid arthritis and premature ageing).

At a time when you are aiming to increase your fertility by optimising your health, anything that may compromise your health should be looked at carefully.

Heavy Toxic Metals

All of these are covered in Section 2 but some of them need to be emphasised now because of their effects on fertility.

Mercury

Mercury is a heavy toxic metal which now contaminates the air, soil and water in many parts of the world. Mercury pollution has been caused by the burning of fossil fuels and the increased use of mercury in industry and agriculture. Traces of mercury can be found in pesticides, dental fillings, and in fish (especially tuna). The saying 'mad as a hatter' came about because hatters used to polish top hats with mercury and many of them were poisoned by it. It is extremely toxic and can affect fertility.

Female dental assistants, for instance, who are exposed to mercury through the amalgam fillings they handle, have been found to be less fertile than female dental assistants who do not come into contact with the metal.[49] And women dentists, it is claimed, have a higher rate of miscarriage.[50]

There are real concerns about the impact of mercury on male fertility, following research in Hong Kong where people eat a lot of fish and shellfish containing minute and supposedly safe quantities of the metal. Here, scientists found a significant link between the level of mercury in hair and male subfertility. Eating mercury-contaminated fish over a number of years stopped sperm development in many Hong Kong men.[51]

Mercury seemed to be one factor in the case of Teresa and her partner.

Case History

Teresa and her partner conceived easily but she was diagnosed with a blighted ovum when she was 10 weeks pregnant and had to have a D&C. Teresa had deficiencies of both zinc and selenium and her partner was low in magnesium with above average levels of mercury. He told me that as a child he had played with mercury. Mercury is an unusual metal, in that it is liquid at room temperature and forms small balls as it flows. Over the four months of the Preconception Plan (see Section 6) they both took specific nutritional supplements to correct their deficiencies and Teresa's partner had extra antioxidants and support for his liver in order to eliminate the mercury. They now have a baby boy.

Lead

Lead is a heavy toxic metal which is naturally present in the earth but we get a high exposure to this metal from lead pipes.

Lead was used in the past to induce an abortion,[52] and severe lead intoxication has been shown to result in infertility and miscarriage.[53] It could be argued that these problems are due to lead poisoning and that most of us are not exposed to such high levels. However, women who just live in lead-polluted areas have also shown a greater risk of miscarriages.[54]

According to a 1991 study, of all the toxic metals, lead seems to pose the greatest threat to male fertility.[55] Research shows that it can reduce the sperm count, increase malformed sperm and make the sperm more sluggish.

Cadmium

This is an inorganic poison present in tobacco smoke which accumulates in the body. It blocks nutrients like zinc – which, as you will see in Section 2, is absolutely crucial for both male and female fertility.

Copper

Copper can be both toxic and essential, depending on how much you are exposed to it. Your body absorbs copper from water pipes, contraceptive coils, swimming pools and jewellery. Copper tends to increase its concentration in the body after any hormonal treatment, such as the Pill or fertility drugs. Copper and zinc are antagonistic which means that if you have too much copper, your zinc levels can be reduced. As zinc is so vital for fertility for both of you, it is important that your copper levels are kept in check.

Zinc deficiency and high lead levels were certainly factors for Janet and her partner.

Case History

Janet, 38, had a miscarriage at 12 weeks before she came to see me. Her nutritional analysis showed that she was low in calcium, selenium and zinc, and had higher than normal levels of lead. Her partner, 34, had low levels of selenium and zinc and very high levels of lead. I felt it was important that they both got themselves back into optimum health by following the Four-Month Preconception Plan outlined in Section 6, before they tried again, in order to try and prevent another miscarriage. I recommended appropriate supplements for their deficiencies, as well as antioxidants like vitamin C to help eliminate the lead from their bodies.

Janet and her partner waited until their mineral and lead levels were back to normal and then conceived and gave birth to a healthy baby boy.

CHAPTER 5

Occupational Hazards

Certain kinds of work may be linked with reduced fertility for both partners. This is backed up by substantial research.

For example, professional drivers spend long hours sitting which can
result in a lower sperm count and higher numbers of abnormal sperm.[56]

Likewise, welders exposed to intense heat may have reduced quantity and
quality of sperm.[57] In the same way, firefighters face intense heat, and they
are also exposed to a large variety of chemicals which affect their fertility.
Indeed, any man who works in a hot environment (such as a foundry or
bakery) could find that his sperm production decreases.

Agricultural workers exposed to pesticides and other chemicals have low
sperm counts. Research also shows that their partners have a high rate of
miscarriages.[58] In 1991, 1,500 men in Costa Rica became sterile after being
exposed to a pesticide used to treat bananas.[59] Other pesticides, such as
DBCP (dibromochloropropane), have caused changes in sperm counts,
some of which were reversible after exposure had stopped.[60] Women
exposed to pesticides can have problems conceiving and an increase in miscarriages.[61]

Healthcare workers can be exposed to waste anaesthetic gases, ethylene
oxide, cytostatic drugs, mercury and X-rays. And, as we have already seen,
dentists and their assistants experience fertility problems due to the mercury in amalgam fillings.

Painters and printers are exposed to solvents and pigments which can
affect male fertility.

Women who are exposed to chemicals and heavy metals often have
problems with their menstrual cycle, experiencing hormone imbalances
and miscarriages, while taking longer to get pregnant.[62]

Problems with fertility can occur if you or your partner work with lead (used to make storage batteries), radiation, pesticides and/or solvents. For example, workers in drycleaners and hairdressers come into contact with a wide range of chemicals.

In 1997 the *Lancet*, the leading medical journal, published a whole range of occupations and their implications for fertility. Agents toxic to sperm included inorganic mercury, dibromochloropropane, ethylene dibromide, ethylene glycol ethers, chloropropene and carbon disulfide. Certain other occupational risks were found, including heat, strenuous work, ionising radiation, exposure to lead, antineoplastic agents, waste anaesthetic gases, ethylene oxide, methyl mercury, polychlorinated biphenyls and carbon monoxide.[63]

Visual Display Units

Like televisions, VDUs produce a range of electromagnetic radiation frequencies, including ultraviolet, infrared, microwave, radio frequency and extra low frequency (ELF). Even though so many workers, male and female, now sit in front of a screen all day, surprisingly little is known about the impact of VDUs on health and fertility.

The Health and Safety Executive, the UK's main workers' watchdog, found no evidence of an increased miscarriage risk among VDU operatives in a 1992 survey. But other studies point to dangers.

The length of time spent at the computer may be the key. One study found that women who spent more than 20 hours a week in front of the screen had twice as many miscarriages as non-VDU workers.[64] But under 20 hours there was no increased risk.[65] Researchers have also found that not only are miscarriages correlated to the amount of time spent on a VDU but also the same for premature births and stillbirths. Out of those spending up to 6 hours a day at a computer 66 per cent had a problem relating to either a miscarriage, premature birth or stillbirth compared to only 25 per cent for those women spending one hour a day on a VDU.[66]

A number of studies on women VDU workers have also considered stress as a contributing factor to fertility problems. Working at a screen means that women can be sitting in the same position for long hours, doing repetitive work, and often under time pressure.

Stress

Doctors are divided over the importance of stress in infertility and yet studies have shown that it can affect a man's fertility to the point where not only the count is reduced but also the quality of the sperm, with abnormal sperm and decreased motility.[67]

Stress can also affect a man's hormone balance, lowering his levels of testosterone and luteinising hormone.[68]

The release of the stress hormone prolactin in response to a crisis can affect a woman's ability to conceive and in extreme cases can stop her ovulating. It seems to be nature's way of protecting women from getting pregnant at a time when they would find it hard to cope. Women going through a bereavement or other kind of trauma for instance can stop having periods altogether.[69]

Couples trying for a baby often experience high levels of stress, particularly if medical intervention is required. The longer it takes, of course, the more anxious you may become – and the more chance there is of stress inhibiting your fertility. A number of studies show that if a woman becomes totally obsessed with having a baby she may release eggs which are not mature enough to be fertilised.[70]

There are many anecdotes concerning couples who have given up fertility investigations, put their names down for adoption, and then found themselves pregnant. One lady I saw gave up work to have a baby and got so bored that she decided to find another job and then got pregnant. Other women may find that the stress of the job they are doing may be affecting their fertility. We are all so different and what affects one person may not trouble another – 'one man's meat is another man's poison'.

Many couples find that they conceive on holiday when they are relaxed and have forgotten about all their domestic worries. Infertility is clearly a multi-factorial problem, which is why this book looks at all the possibilities, not only the physical aspects (such as hormones and nutrition) but also the psychological and emotional side.

The next section explains how you and your partner can help improve your own fertility.

SECTION 2

WHAT *YOU* CAN DO TO HELP YOURSELF

❀

The previous section described the factors that can affect your fertility. This section tells you what you can do to increase your fertility and chances of conceiving. Some of the recommendations directly affect your fertility, others can prevent a miscarriage. They will all have an impact on your general health which will in turn boost your fertility. The benefits are enormous – not only in helping you conceive but in improving your whole lifestyle and helping you to have a healthy pregnancy and a healthy baby.

If you are planning to go for IVF or another fertility treatment the recommendations here will dramatically increase the chance of these procedures being successful.

This has been borne out by work at the Reproductive Healthcare Clinic in St John's Wood, London. Results of treatment there showed that women between 32 and 43 years old who underwent 40 cycles of assisted conception achieved an astonishingly successful pregnancy rate of 50 per cent, compared to the standard 15 per cent.

These remarkable results were achieved by a combination of conventional and complementary medicine. While the couples were being medically investigated by Reproductive Healthcare's director consultant gynaecologist and specialist in reproductive medicine, Mr Talha Shawaf, and treated in collaboration with one of London's leading fertility centres, they also came to see me and had full nutritional analysis, lifestyle recommendations and a supplement programme for the months leading up to treatment.

By having 'the best of both worlds' they achieved a 50 per cent pregnancy rate. This shows that conventional and complementary medicine need not be mutually exclusive. They can be used very successfully together – all it requires is open-mindedness on the part of both the conventional and the complementary practitioner, who can learn from each other, and open-mindedness on your part too. You have nothing to lose and everything to gain, as Jill and her partner discovered.

Case History

Before coming to see me, Jill and her partner, both in their early thirties, had been trying to conceive for two years. Jill's blood tests showed abnormal reproductive hormone levels and her scan showed that one ovary was not functioning and that the other one had multiple cysts, a symptom of polycystic ovary syndrome (PCOS).

Her partner had had a number of sperm tests with conflicting results, and a post-coital test (see page 142) had shown no sperm in the sample. They both had stressful jobs and worked long hours.

Before the diagnosis of PCOS she had been treated for eight months with clomiphene citrate, and they had had one unsuccessful IUI attempt. They had already decided to go for IVF treatment by the time they came to see me, so the aim was to get them as healthy as possible before the treatment started. From the mineral analysis, I could see a number of deficiencies so these were corrected before the IVF cycle started. They were successful on their first IVF attempt and now have a lovely baby girl.

CHAPTER 6

Timing When You Have Intercourse

Hormonal Harmony

Nature has designed your reproductive system to work in harmony, each hormone dependent on the other and all working together as a whole system. Any imbalance in any part of this delicate process will affect the production of hormones and with it the chances of conceiving or staying pregnant once fertilisation has occurred. It does not take much to upset the balance; but simple changes in diet and lifestyle can restore it. By getting yourself into optimum health you increase the chances of conceiving because your whole reproductive system will operate more efficiently.

Let's first look at the hormones step by step, over one cycle, to see how they work:

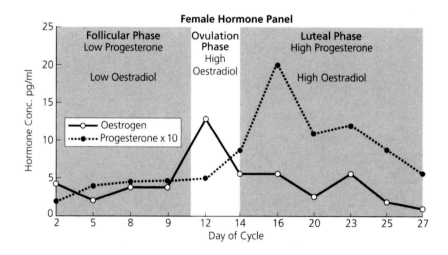

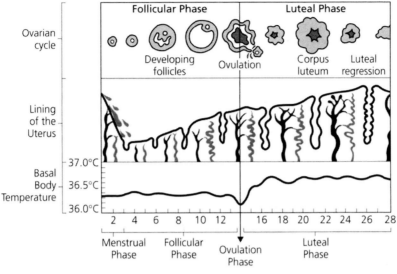

A Normal Female Hormonal Cycle

1. At the beginning of the menstrual cycle (first day of the period), **FSH (follicle stimulating hormone)** is released from the pituitary gland.

2. The **FSH** stimulates a group of follicles to grow on the surface of the ovary.

3. Over the next two weeks (the follicular phase of the cycle), the eggs grow and mature and **oestrogen** produced by the ovary keeps increasing.

4. As the **oestrogen** levels increase, the pituitary gland decreases its production of **FSH**, and **LH (luteinising hormone)** production is then triggered. Fertile alkaline mucus is produced in the cervix ready to keep the sperm alive and to speed its transport.

5. As the **LH** surges, the mature egg (usually only one) is released from the follicle (ovulation) and enters the fallopian tube.

6. The empty follicle becomes the corpus luteum which produces **progesterone**. This is the second half of the cycle (the luteal phase).

7. The fertilised egg stays in the fallopian tube for seven days. On the seventh day after fertilisation (i.e. approximately day 21 of the cycle), the egg (which is now a developing embryo) develops chorionic villi

which are special protrusions on its surface to enable it to implant in the womb lining.

8. The chorionic villi produce a hormone called human **chorionic gonadotrophin (hCG)** which means that the corpus luteum continues to increase in size and produce more **progesterone**, thus maintaining the pregnancy. (**hCG** is the hormone that is picked up by a pregnancy testing kit.)

The timing of all this is crucial. It is vital that the journey through the fallopian tube takes around seven days. If it is shorter then the fertilised egg could arrive in the womb before it is able to embed itself in the lining and die. If the journey takes much longer than seven days then the fertilised egg could embed itself in the fallopian tube instead, causing an ectopic or tubal pregnancy which can be life-threatening for the woman.

What Happens in a Monthly Cycle?

As you can see, the monthly cycle is governed by the reproductive hormones, the main ones being oestrogen, progesterone, follicle stimulating hormone (FSH) and luteinising hormone (LH).

WHAT ARE HORMONES?

Hormones are chemical messengers and the word comes from a Greek word meaning 'urge on'. Carried in the bloodstream, they trigger activity in different organs and body parts. The reproductive hormones control the monthly cycle and help to maintain pregnancy.

At the beginning of each menstrual cycle, the oestrogen and progesterone levels are low and the follicle stimulating hormone (FSH) is produced by the pituitary gland in the brain which controls the whole endocrine (hormone) system.

This begins the process of ovulation by stimulating the ovaries to produce the hormone, oestrogen.

> ### OESTROGEN
>
> Oestrogen is not just one hormone but several grouped together.
> But for the sake of clarity I will use the term oestrogen to include
> all of them. Oestrogen is the key hormone responsible for a
> woman maturing from childhood to adulthood. It causes the
> breasts to develop and produces the characteristic feminine shape.

The lining of the womb (uterus) starts to thicken each month as it prepares
to receive a fertilised egg.

Ovulation

The oestrogen level continues to rise until the middle of the month when
the pituitary gland produces luteinising hormone (LH) which triggers
ovulation. The egg (ovum) is then released from a follicle in the ovary and
passes down the fallopian tube.

After ovulation, the ovaries produce progesterone, which prevents any further ovulation taking place in that cycle. If fertilisation does not occur, the
lining of the womb breaks down and menstruation takes place. At the same
time there is a dramatic and rapid fall in the levels of oestrogen and progesterone and, with this drop in hormone levels, the cycle starts all over again.

Fertilisation

When fertilisation occurs the egg implants itself into the thick and nour-
ishing wall of the womb, where it begins to develop.

Fertilisation usually takes place in the fallopian tube. Once this has happened, the empty follicle, which released the egg, forms the corpus luteum
which produces progesterone.

In each menstrual cycle, a group of about 20 follicles containing the
developing eggs grows on the surface of the ovary. Generally only the
biggest follicle continues to develop, which is why humans usually only
have one baby at a time.

> **PROGESTERONE**
>
> Progesterone is an important hormone in fertility because it maintains the womb lining during the second half of the cycle, in readiness for a fertilised egg. It is also responsible for maintaining the pregnancy.

Getting Your Timing Right

The bottom part of the womb, the cervix, changes quite dramatically during the menstrual cycle according to the hormones being produced. Understanding and recognising these changes is one of the most important ways you can pinpoint the best time to have intercourse in order to conceive.

The mucus-secreting glands (crypts) which line the cervical canal produce mucus continuously but this fluid undergoes important changes during the menstrual cycle. During the first half of the cycle (the follicular phase), the mucus is thick and sticky. It forms a plug over the cervix, which stops semen entering. It also makes the vagina acid, which can kill off sperm within a few hours.

About three to four days before ovulation, as oestrogen levels increase, the mucus becomes clear and stretchy and the amount increases. Surrounded by this fertile mucus, sperm can live for up to seven days.[71]

So it is possible to have intercourse on a Monday and actually conceive on a Friday! This fertile mucus turns the vaginal fluids alkaline, keeping sperm alive. It also provides nourishment for the sperm, in the form of increased amounts of sugar, amino acids, salt and water.

The other intriguing aspect of this fertile mucus is that it forms 'swimming lanes' (or canals) through which the sperm can pass quickly. It also seems to act as a filter, allowing the healthy sperm to travel forward but effectively trapping the abnormal sperm (there are always some abnormal sperm in semen) and blocking their passage. Once ovulation has taken place and progesterone increases, the mucus again becomes thick and sticky (infertile mucus), protecting the cervix from sperm and also from any foreign bodies.

Checking Your Fertility

Since the egg can only survive for up to 24 hours and the sperm can live for seven days in alkaline mucus, there is only a short window of time each month in which you can conceive.

Some women only produce fertile mucus for a day or two a month so it is vital to know when it is happening. It is all too easy to have intercourse at the wrong time of the month or not frequently enough at the right time. Here's how you can identify your crucial fertile period for yourself:

WARNING

Note that you will not be able to use this test if you have thrush or some other vaginal discharge because it will not be possible to see the changes in your cervical mucus. Any such problems should be treated before you try for a baby.

- After passing urine, blot your vaginal mucus with white toilet paper.
- Lightly apply a finger to the mucus on the toilet paper and then pull gently away to test its ability to stretch.
- If it feels slippery, like raw egg white, and can stretch between your thumb and first finger up to several inches before it breaks, then it is fertile mucus. If it is sticky or crumbly (a bit like 'school glue') then it is the more acid, infertile mucus. As the mucus changes to fertile mucus, this is a sign that ovulation is about to take place.

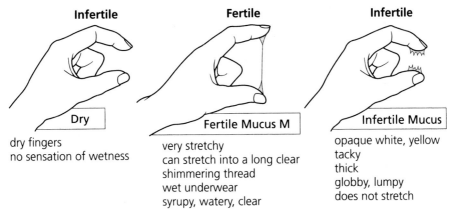

Infertile	Fertile	Infertile
Dry	Fertile Mucus M	Infertile Mucus
dry fingers no sensation of wetness	very stretchy can stretch into a long clear shimmering thread wet underwear syrupy, watery, clear	opaque white, yellow tacky thick globby, lumpy does not stretch

Checking Your Fertility

- Meanwhile, your cervix is also changing. To feel these changes, empty your bladder and wash your hands. Then place your right index finger in your vagina until you can feel your cervix.
- As your period ends, your cervix is located low in your vaginal canal and the opening is closed, giving the feeling of touching the tip of a nose or a small rubber ball. As ovulation approaches and oestrogen levels increase, the cervix moves higher into the vaginal opening, making it more difficult to reach. It also begins to soften and opens, resembling parted lips. This opening and rising helps the sperm to travel into the womb. After ovulation, the cervix lowers again and closes and is blocked with mucus to stop sperm entering.

The best way to take advantage of this window of time is to have inter-course on the first day when you feel wet vaginally and notice that the dis-charge is stretchy. Intercourse should continue every other day while the mucus stays wet and stretchy. Taking a break of 48 hours between inter-course allows time to maximise sperm volume. This is very important.

However, it is also important that this method or the use of ovulation kits (described below) does not take over your lives. For example, I know of a man who was phoned at work by his wife because she had found fertile mucus and wanted him to come home straight away! In situations like this, spontaneity can be lost, the man can feel that he is just viewed as a breeding stud, and both partners can lose the enjoyment of love-making.

Taking Your Temperature

The temperature rise around the middle of the cycle confirms that ovula-tion has taken place, though it cannot predict it in advance. But charting your temperature each day tells you that you are ovulating and when. So this is another way to identify when you are likely to be fertile in future cycles.

If your cycle is regular there should be a temperature rise between days 14 and 16. It is on the days just before this point that you should be at your most fertile. Count the days from the beginning of your last period when you are estimating this. Using this method, you should have intercourse every other day from about day 11 to day 16 even if you are unsure about the mucus changes.

Because the temperature reading has to be the basal body temperature it needs to be measured first thing in the morning. Our normal body temperature rises as the day goes on, so it is important to take it at the same time each day, in order to distinguish between a routine rise and the rise that occurs after ovulation.

To use this method:

- Take your temperature first thing in the morning while you are lying in bed, before you have a drink or go to the toilet. You should wake up and immediately put the thermometer under your tongue.
- The easiest type of thermometer to use is an electronic digital thermometer, now available from most chemists (B-D is a good make), as it registers the temperature within one minute and often has a memory. This can be convenient if you like a lie-in at the weekend. Then you can just set your alarm, take your temperature at 7am, turn the thermometer off when it 'bleeps', and the temperature reading will be stored for later when you can write it down.
- If you are using a mercury thermometer then it must be a special 'ovulation thermometer', as it needs to have an expanded scale. If you can get a Fahrenheit thermometer (either digital or electronic) it will be easier to see the rise in temperature at ovulation.

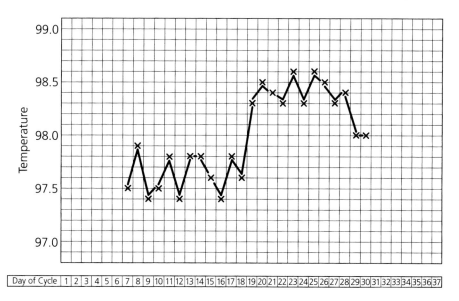

Temperature Change Over One Cycle

• You will need to plot the temperatures on a graph to see the changes over the cycle. Use a different graph for each cycle, counting the first day of your period as day 1. Since most (but by no means all) women have a 28-day cycle, you have to count the actual days and not rely on calendar dates to pinpoint the vital days in the month ahead when you should be at your most fertile.

Remember, however, that many factors can affect your temperature – illness (fever), disturbed nights, travelling across time zones, shift work, alcohol and drugs. So there are now a number of other ways of charting ovulation.

Ovulation Kits

These do-it-yourself kits (such as Clearplan) enable you to predict ovulation by measuring the LH surge in an early morning urine sample. You do this using a specially designed dipstick which changes colour when the levels of LH increase. When your LH surges it is likely that ovulation will occur within the next 24–36 hours, so it is advisable to have intercourse during this time.

The kits are available from most chemists and come with full instructions. They are very easy to use and the instructions tell you when to start testing, depending on the length of your cycle. For example, if you have a 28-day cycle then the first day of testing is day 11. There are usually five dipsticks in a kit and the recommendation is to keep testing until the LH surge is registered, so not all five dipsticks need be used in one cycle.

WARNING

If you have been diagnosed with polycystic ovaries you should not use these kits because the results will be misleading. Polycystic ovaries result in high LH levels which means that, whatever time in the month you are testing, the kit may register positive.

Persona

This device is manufactured by Unipath and has been marketed as a method of contraception. It is a small gadget which uses dipsticks during the month to measure LH changes. The dipsticks are inserted into the device and a green light indicates that it is safe to have intercourse. When there is the possibility of getting pregnant a red light appears and on days when ovulation may be occurring an 'O' appears in one of the display windows.

Used in reverse, to highlight your most fertile time, this device can be very useful. Because it is designed for contraception, it errs on the side of caution which means the red light will come on for slightly longer. Some women find this device easier to use than the usual ovulation kits because it actually signals when the testing should take place in any cycle.

There is no reason why you should not try both, to find out which kind of kit suits you best. The important thing is that you should be able to establish, through testing your mucus and taking your temperature or using a kit, which are the fertile days in your cycle. Getting the timing of intercourse right is one of the most crucial ways to help yourself conceive.

CHAPTER 7

Improving Your Diet

The food you eat has an impact on every cell of your body. This is why a healthy diet is so important, because it really can help you conceive and give birth to a healthy baby. But good nutrition doesn't have to mean giving up all the things you like. It just means being well-informed about food and making the right choices. In fact, once you start following the guidelines below, you may well find that you enjoy food more than you used to, especially when you consider how much good it's doing you. If you find it hard to think of recipes there are plenty of healthy eating cook-books available from bookshops and libraries. These are a great source of inspiration and ideas, and will prove that healthy food can also taste delicious.

Because the dietary and lifestyle changes described in this section of the book take time to have an effect, you and your partner should start putting the advice into practice *at least four months before* you start trying to conceive. That will give you plenty of time to 'spring-clean' your system and correct any nutritional deficiencies. Another reason for this four-month preparation period is that it takes around three months for your partner to produce a new batch of sperm and also three months for your egg to mature, ready for ovulation.

This chapter begins by listing the 'dos and don'ts' of healthy eating, then explains the importance of being the correct weight and balancing your blood sugar level, and finishes with a guide to shopping for healthy food.

What *Should* You Eat?

Essential Fats

Unfortunately fat has got itself a bad name, although it's actually only saturated fats that are harmful. Many women now consciously avoid all fats as a matter of course. But there are some fats which are vital for your health – and your fertility.

These are called essential fatty acids and they are found in foods such as nuts, seeds and oily fish. These essential fats are a vital component of every human cell and the body needs them to balance hormones, insulate nerve cells, keep the skin and arteries supple, and keep itself warm.

Unsaturated fats can be divided into monounsaturated and polyunsaturated fats. Monounsaturated fats are not classed as essential fatty acids. Olive oil is high in these monounsaturated fats, which are thought to lower the risks of heart attacks and other circulatory problems.

Polyunsaturated fats can be split into Omega 6 oils (found in unrefined safflower, corn, sesame and sunflower oils) and Omega 3 oils (found in fish oils and linseed or flax oil). The body makes beneficial prostaglandins (hormone-like regulating substances) from Omega 3 and Omega 6 oils, so that is why they are particularly useful for increasing fertility.

If you are not getting enough of these essential fatty acids, you may notice symptoms such as:

- Dry skin
- Cracked skin on heels or fingertips
- Hair falling out
- Poor wound healing
- Dry, difficult hair
- Dandruff
- Irritability
- Soft or brittle nails
- Allergies
- Fatigue
- Hyperactivity
- Difficulty losing weight
- High blood pressure
- Arthritis
- Pre-menstrual syndrome
- Painful breasts

If you have several of the above symptoms they may also be due to thyroid imbalance which can also affect your fertility, so it is worth checking with your doctor.

ESSENTIAL FATTY ACID SUPPLEMENTS

Most of us don't eat enough essential fats, so when you are trying to maximise your fertility it's a good idea to add them to your diet in supplement form (see page 84). Research has shown the benefits of supplementing with essential fatty acids during pregnancy to avoid low birthweight and also the advantages to the growing baby in terms of brain development.

To achieve a satisfactory intake of essential fatty acids, have a daily handful of nuts or use a salad dressing made with a good-quality nut or seed oil. You can also eat oily fish (such as mackerel or sardines) and take an essential fatty acid supplement (see page 84).

CHOOSING AND USING OILS

Oils can easily get damaged so you need to take care when choosing, storing and using them. If oils are over-heated, left in sunlight or re-used after cooking, they are open to attack by free radicals (which have been linked to cancer, coronary heart disease, rheumatoid arthritis and premature ageing).

To avoid the formation of free radicals, always choose cold-pressed unrefined nut or seed oils or extra-virgin olive oil. A number of supermarkets now have organic oils. Unfortunately, non-organic standard supermarket oils are manufactured and extracted using chemicals and heat. This destroys the quality of the oil and its nutritional content. Store your oil away from sunlight and do not be tempted to re-use it after cooking.

Do not fry polyunsaturated fats, as they can become oxidised when heated. Use olive oil or butter for frying. Monounsaturated olive oil is less likely to create free radicals and butter will not because it is a saturated fat. Reduce the cooking temperature to minimise oxidation. Keep all fats to a minimum when frying. Try to bake or grill instead.

Fibre

We need fibre to keep our bowels healthy and prevent constipation but fibre is also vital for our fertility.

The fibre contained in wholegrains, fruit and vegetables reduces excess oestrogen levels, clearing out old hormone residues. It does this by preventing oestrogens that have been excreted in the bile from being reabsorbed back into the blood.

Studies have shown that women who eat a vegetarian diet excrete three times more 'old', detoxified oestrogens than women who also eat meat. The meat-eaters also reabsorb more oestrogen. So, for both men and women aiming to keep their reproductive systems in optimum balance, it makes sense to ensure that you are getting enough fibre in your diet.

Contrary to popular belief, the best way to do this is *not* to add bran to your food. Whatever you may have read or heard about its benefits, bran can actually block the absorption of vital nutrients such as iron, zinc, calcium and magnesium. It is much better to eat it in its natural form (as wholegrains) instead.

To increase your fibre intake, you need to eat plenty of fresh fruit and vegetables (cooked and raw), wholegrains (brown rice, wholemeal bread, oats, wholegrain crackers and wholemeal pasta), beans, nuts and seeds.

You should also avoid refined carbohydrates (such as cakes, white bread and biscuits, and anything containing white flour and sugar). Don't be tempted to eat bran on its own or when added or made into breakfast cereal.

It is important for your bowels to work efficiently so that 'old' hormones can be quickly excreted and also so that food does not end up putrefying (which it may do if it stays in your bowel too long). Proper bowel function also helps you get rid of chemicals, pesticides, heavy toxic metals and other toxins that can affect your fertility.

I have found that even patients diagnosed with high lead levels, caused by daily commuting to work through London, soon start to get rid of the excess lead once they are on a healthy, high-fibre diet.

HELP FOR CONSTIPATION

What can you use instead of bran? First try increasing your intake of fresh fruit and vegetables. If you need extra help then either sprinkle 1 tablespoon of linseeds onto your breakfast cereal in the mornings or soak 1 tablespoon of linseeds in a small amount of water and swallow. Vitamin C can also be used to help soften stools. Try taking 1,000mg per day, and increase by 500mg at a time until your stools are manageable, soft and comfortable.

Complex Carbohydrates

Carbohydrates include sugars and starches. They are an important source of energy and are all eventually broken down in your body into the simple sugar, glucose. There are two types of carbohydrate – complex and simple. Complex carbohydrates include grains (such as wheat, rye, oats, rice, barley and maize), beans and pulses (such as lentils, chickpeas and kidney beans), and vegetables. Simple carbohydrates include white and brown sugar, honey, fruit and fruit juice.

To optimise your health, you should eat plenty of unrefined complex carbohydrates. This means choosing brown wholemeal bread, brown rice and brown pasta, instead of the refined white versions which have been stripped of essential vitamins, minerals, trace elements and valuable fibre content. (In order to digest these refined foods your body has to use its own vitamins and minerals, thus depleting your stores.)

Simple carbohydrates, in the form of fruit and dried fruit, certainly have a place in a healthy, balanced diet. But it's important, for your health and fertility, to maintain a steady blood sugar level (see page 61). For this reason, you should avoid sugar, honey and undiluted fruit juice, which can all produce a sudden rise in blood sugar, followed by a sudden fall.

Soya

Soya is being studied extensively around the world for its effectiveness in lowering cholesterol and preventing cardiovascular disease. It also appears to have an important role to play in balancing male and female sex hormones. Scientists believe that hormonal imbalance and over-exposure to chemicals that have oestrogen-like qualities may be one reason for the rapid increase in breast and prostate cancers over the last couple of decades. Crucially, this hormonal dysfunction and overload are also implicated in the menstrual and reproductive problems that affect fertility.

Soya is classed as a phyto-oestrogen, which means that it contains substances that act like hormones. These phyto-oestrogens fit into oestrogen receptors in the breast and block them, effectively shielding the body from exposure to oestrogen which is believed to be one of the major causes of breast cancer. Studies of Japanese women, who traditionally eat a great deal of soya, suggest that it may protect them from this disease.[72]

Oestrogen is not only implicated in breast cancer but is also believed to play a part in causing other problems like endometriosis, fibroids, and heavy and/or long periods – all of which can affect female fertility.

Some women have problems conceiving because the second half of their menstrual cycle, just after ovulation, is shorter than it should be. This 'luteal phase defect', as it is known, means that there is not enough progesterone at the right time to maintain a pregnancy. Scientists have found that if they add soya to a woman's diet it can lengthen the cycle by 2.5 days.[73]

For all these reasons, it's well worth adding soya to your diet – perhaps in the form of soya milk and tofu (soya beancurd, often used in Oriental stir-fried dishes). However, you need to ensure that the soya used to manufacture these products is not genetically modified (see page 55), so buy organic.

Summary

So, for optimum health during this four-month preparation period, you should eat plenty of:

- Essential fats (nuts, seeds and oily fish)
- High-fibre foods (fruit, vegetables, wholegrains, beans, nuts and seeds)
- Complex carbohydrates (wholegrains, beans, pulses and vegetables)
- Non-GM organic soya

What Shouldn't *You Eat or Drink?*

Caffeine

Caffeine comes in many forms besides tea and coffee. It is also in colas, other soft drinks, chocolate, and pain-relieving medication such as headache remedies, so it is easy to end up with an excess of caffeine.

HOW MUCH CAFFEINE IS IN YOUR DIET?	
One cup of ground coffee	115mg
One 125g (4oz) bar of dark chocolate	80mg
One cup of instant coffee	65mg
Two painkiller tablets	60mg
One cup of tea	50mg
One can of cola	40mg
One 125g (4oz) bar of milk chocolate	20mg
One cup of drinking chocolate	3mg
One cup of decaffeinated coffee	3mg

Tea contains tannin as well as caffeine. Tannin binds important minerals and prevents their absorption in the digestive tract. This means that, if you drink tea at mealtimes, you could eat a nutritious meal, and take vitamins and minerals, and yet waste these vital nutrients by excreting them unabsorbed.

Caffeine is a stimulant but, because tea and coffee are socially acceptable, we tend to forget their addictive properties. If you are a frequent coffee drinker and suddenly stop, you may well experience quite dramatic withdrawal symptoms, including headaches, nausea, tiredness and depression.

Some hospitals have now discovered that certain post-operative symptoms are not caused by the effects of the anaesthetic (as previously thought), but by caffeine withdrawal. Before a general anaesthetic patients are asked not to eat or drink for a number of hours and by the time they come round from the operation the caffeine withdrawal symptoms have started.

If you suddenly go from drinking three cups of coffee a day to none the next day, the withdrawal effects can be horrendous, including headaches and shaking. It's therefore much better to cut down slowly over a few weeks. Perhaps first substitute decaffeinated for half of your total cups per day, then gradually change over to all decaffeinated. You can then gradually substitute other drinks, such as herbal teas and grain coffees. (You will eventually have to eliminate decaffeinated coffee too, since it contains other unhelpful stimulants even with the caffeine removed.)

If you are finding it hard to give up, remind yourself that it may be stopping you getting pregnant. There is plenty of evidence:

- Drinking as little as one cup of coffee a day decreases your fertility and can halve your chance of conceiving.[74]
- Caffeine delays conception. Several studies have shown that women who drink coffee find it three times as difficult to conceive within a year as those not drinking it.[75]
- Men don't escape the effects of caffeine either. Problems with sperm health (such as count, motility and abnormalities) seem to increase, the more cups of coffee men drink each day.[76] This may be partly because caffeine has a diuretic effect (making you want to pass more urine), and this can flush out vital nutrient and trace elements that are important for fertility, such as zinc.

The message from all these studies is that if you want to increase your fertility, and reduce the time it takes you to get pregnant, then drinks and food containing caffeine need to be eliminated altogether.

Saturated Fat

A diet high in saturated fat is known to stimulate oestrogen production which can compromise fertility.[77] Animal products are the main source of saturated fats, so you need to reduce your intake of meat, eggs and dairy produce.

Meat

Beef, pork, lamb and game should, in my opinion, be omitted completely. Apart from the hormones pumped into the animals, red meat has been linked to illnesses such as bowel cancer and diverticulitis (a condition in which parts of the colon protrude and get inflamed).

In 1997 the Government's Department of Health Committee on Medical Aspects of Food and Nutrition Policy (COMA) took the rare step of publishing a report entitled *Nutritional Aspects of the Development of Cancer*, which suggested a possible link between the consumption of red meat and bowel cancer. It suggested that intakes at or above the current average of around 90g (3.2oz) per day should be reduced. When you consider that an average portion of bacon is 45g (1.6oz), while just two pork sausages weigh approximately 100g (3.5oz), it makes you realise how easy it is to eat far too much red meat.

The saturated fats in red meat and poultry produce a hormone called prostaglandin PGE2 which is highly inflammatory. It can cause swelling and pain, including period pains, and may worsen the symptoms of endometriosis. It has also been linked to the spread of endometrial tissue which can be a major cause of infertility.

Chicken can also be a source of salmonella infection. Buy organic chicken if you can, and cook it thoroughly to kill off any harmful bacteria.

Eggs

Choose organic free-range eggs which have been produced without the use of growth promoters, antibiotics or hormones. That way you are reducing your intake of chemicals which can have a direct effect on fertility.

Dairy Products

Farmers give their cattle antibiotics to speed their growth as well as hormones to increase the supply of milk per cow. A generation ago, an individual cow would produce approximately 9 litres (2 gallons) of milk per day; now it yields 56 litres (12 gallons) per day. These hormones must surely end up in the milk. At a time when you are trying to boost your fertility you don't want excess hormones coming from outside, as it is crucial that your own and your partner's hormones are within the normal range.

So, if you are buying dairy products, again buy organic in order to reduce your intake of chemicals and hormones. Organic dairy produce is available in most supermarkets.

Of all dairy foods, yogurt containing the culture *Lactobacillus acidophilus*, which is a natural inhabitant of our gut, is the most beneficial. When yogurts are heat treated they lose their original culture so no benefit is gained from eating them. Buy natural yogurt that is 'live' and organic. This can be marketed in different ways, so read the labels carefully. 'Bio' usually means 'live', and 'bio' yogurts will contain a culture like Lactobacillus. Avoid fruit yogurts which can have a very high sugar content.

Taking *Lactobacillus acidophilus* as a supplement (available in capsule form from all good healthfood shops) can also be beneficial, as it lowers the level of the enzymes which reabsorb 'old' hormones. Each month your body should eliminate all the hormones it doesn't need. But, unfortunately, it sometimes reabsorbs some of them, creating an imbalance. This imbalance can affect your fertility so anything that helps your body to excrete more efficiently is useful.

HEALTH RISKS OF SATURATED FATS

1. Becoming overweight
The more saturated a fat becomes, the harder it is to digest. So it ends up being stored in the body. Butter, coconut oil and palm oil are the saturated fats most easily assimilated by the body, so they are less harmful. Fat from beef, lamb and pork are the hardest to digest because they are hard at body temperature. And being overweight reduces fertility (see page 61).

2. Blocking nutrients
Saturated fats also interfere with your body's absorption of the essential fatty acids which are vital for health and fertility. Trans fatty acids, often contained in fried foods and in margarines under the name 'hydrogenated fats', are the biggest culprit and should always be avoided.

Margarine versus butter

Hydrogenated vegetable oil is listed in the ingredients of most margarines and also many fast foods, crisps, biscuits and crackers. The process of hydrogenation changes the essential unsaturated fats contained in the food into trans fatty acids which have been linked to problems with absorption of essential fats and an increased risk of heart attack.[78]

So I would recommend using moderate amounts of organic butter (most supermarkets now sell it) or unhydrogenated margarine (obtainable from healthfood shops) rather than ordinary margarine. Although margarine is manufactured from polyunsaturated fats it is made into a solid form through hydrogenation. Because these trans fats are not natural in such high levels and have a plastic-like quality, your body has great difficulty getting rid of them. Why put yourself under extra pressure to deal with a substance that you do not really need to eat? It's better to make things easy for your body so that it functions efficiently and, in doing so, has the resources to heal itself and increase your fertility.

Semen is rich in prostaglandins which are produced from essential fatty acids so it is also important for men to avoid trans fatty acids. It is thought that the prostaglandins help to make the sperm motile and are crucial for their survival.[79]

Alcohol

Both you and your partner need to eliminate alcohol (see page 13). If your infertility is caused by problems such as polycystic ovaries, fibroids or endometriosis, alcohol can compromise the efficient functioning of your liver and make it less able to get rid of excess circulating hormones. Alcohol will also stop you absorbing essential nutrients like zinc which are crucial for fertility.

Genetically Modified Foods

We know that the fertility of animals feeding on genetically modified foods can be reduced, so it is only common sense for you to eliminate these foods, as best you can, from your diet. We do not yet know the long-term health risks of GM foods but anything that may compromise good health needs to be avoided when you are aiming to increase your chances of conceiving.

What Are GM Foods?

Genes are a set of coded instructions, made from DNA, which control physical and behavioural characteristics such as hair colour. Genetic modification means that genes from other species can be introduced into a particular plant, usually to make it more resistant to pests, viruses, weedkillers or other hazards. For instance, it is now possible to buy a tomato which contains a fish gene to boost its frost resistance. The gene is from a flounder because they survive well in cold water. This same flounder gene has also been introduced into salmon which could be on the market in two years time. In the cold dark days of winter a salmon stops eating and growing but adding a flounder gene keeps them eating all year round, speeding up their growth rate by 400 per cent. This kind of 'tampering with nature' explains why GM foods have been called 'Frankenstein foods'.

What Are The Risks?

There are worries that GM foods will make various diseases resistant to the antibiotics which have saved millions of us from death in the last few decades.

This is because, when genes are transferred in the lab, marker genes are transferred along with the DNA. This enables scientists to identify which cells have become modified. Usually a gene for antibiotic resistance is used as a marker. The British Medical Association (BMA) fears that resistance to antibiotics might transfer to animals or humans and leave patients vulnerable to diseases such as meningitis. For example, genetically modified maize contains a marker gene which passes on resistance to ampicillin, an important antibiotic used to treat bronchitis, ear infections and urinary tract infections in humans. Some urinary tract infections can impair fertility so we need the medical ammunition to deal with these infections.

The BMA has issued a report, called *The Impact of Genetic Modification on Agriculture, Food and Health*, and has called for studies to see whether these foods could damage our immune system or cause birth defects.

It is also possible that the DNA from our food could be transferred to the natural bacteria in the human gut, creating lethal substances and a whole generation of new diseases which won't be killed off by antibiotics.

How Can You Avoid GM Foods?

Soya is probably the best-known genetically modified food. Up to 60 per cent of processed foods contain soya, including bread, biscuits, pizza and baby food. Lecithin, contained in many foods, is also made from soya. Just what proportion of that 60 per cent is now genetically modified we do not know, but we can probably assume that it is quite considerable. Other genetically modified foods on sale in the UK are maize, tomato paste and cheese containing chymosin (a genetically modified rennet used to harden the cheese).

Since September 1998, manufacturers have been obliged to label products containing genetically modified DNA. However, this labelling only applies to genetically modified soya and maize (corn) products and only where protein or DNA can be detected in the final product by laboratory screening. Foods containing soya oil, refined starches, and additives (such as emulsifiers and lecithins) are excluded. Greenpeace estimate this means that 90 per cent of foods containing genetically modified products are unlabelled. Since the latter part of 1999, because of public opposition to GM foods, supermarkets have been claiming that they have less than 1 per cent GM foods on their shelves and they are trying to go lower than that.

Genetic engineering involves manipulating the basic DNA of a plant or animal. This happens naturally in evolution of course, but with nature in charge the process normally takes hundreds if not thousands of years. It is this process which ensures that the fittest of the species survive. But the gene manipulation that humans are now tinkering with bypasses evolution, and we don't know as yet what the price will be. In order to smuggle these new genes across the species barrier, scientists use infectious agents (viruses and bacteria). Then the antibiotic-resistant genes are used as genetic markers to allow the scientists to track the movements of these new genes. In one instance a nut gene was inserted into a soya bean and people with allergies to nuts became allergic to the soya milk. This would have posed a very serious risk for anyone with a nut allergy who would have had no idea that the soya milk contained a nut gene.

Even the scientists disagree violently as to the value and dangers of genetically modified foods. So the only sensible thing to do is to try to avoid them when you shop for food.

The Vegetarian Society has announced that, from August 1999, all foods bearing the 'V' symbol will have to be free from genetically modified products. Provamel, the market leader for soya products in the UK, have stated that their foods are free from genetically modified material and have implemented a system to trace the soya from seed to final production. Also, at the moment, if a food is labelled organic it is not genetically modified.

My advice is to avoid genetically modified foods where possible by buying organic and reading the labels. If we as consumers consciously do not buy these foods then eventually there may not be a market for them.

Summary

For optimum health during this preparation period, you should:

- Eliminate alcohol and caffeine (coffee, tea, fizzy drinks, chocolate and caffeine-containing headache remedies).
- Reduce your intake of saturated fat (meat, eggs and dairy produce); and, when you do eat these foods, try to make sure they are organic.
- Avoid genetically modified foods by checking labels carefully and buying organic.

Your Weight

Your ability to conceive is significantly affected by what you weigh. You can make some very simple changes here to increase your fertility.

Calculating Your Body Mass Index (BMI)

Being the right weight for your height is very important. The easiest way to measure this is by means of the Body Mass Index (BMI) which identifies the percentage of body tissue which is actually fat. The amount of fat is important for fertility because we produce oestrogen from fat cells.

Your BMI is the ratio of your height to your weight and is calculated as follows: BMI = your weight in kg divided by the square of your height in metres. For example, if my weight is 63.5kg (10 stone) and my height is 1.68m (5ft 6in), my BMI is $63.5 \div 1.68 \times 1.68 = 22.5$.

WHAT DOES YOUR BMI MEAN?

Under 20: underweight
20–25: normal
25–30: overweight
30–40: obese
Over 40: dangerously obese

A BMI of 30 would indicate a person around 16kg (2½ stone) overweight.

stones	ft	4.10	4.11	5.0	5.1	5.2	5.3	5.4	5.5	5.6	5.7	5.8	5.9	5.10	5.11
	cms	147	150	152	155	158	160	163	165	168	170	173	175	178	180
stones	kgs														
6.11	43	20	19	19	18	17	17	16	16	15	15	14	14	14	13
6.13	44	20	20	19	18	18	17	17	16	16	15	15	14	14	14
7.1	45	21	20	19	19	18	18	17	17	16	16	15	15	14	14
7.3	46	21	20	20	19	18	18	17	17	16	16	15	15	15	14
7.6	47	22	21	20	20	19	18	18	17	17	16	16	15	15	15
7.8	48	22	21	21	20	19	19	18	18	17	17	16	16	15	15
7.10	49	23	22	21	20	20	19	18	18	17	17	16	16	15	15
7.12	50	23	22	22	21	20	20	19	18	18	17	17	16	16	15
8	51	24	23	22	21	20	20	19	19	18	18	17	17	16	16
8.3	52	24	23	23	22	21	20	20	19	18	18	17	17	16	16
8.5	53	25	24	23	22	21	21	20	19	19	18	18	17	17	16
8.7	54	25	24	23	22	22	21	20	20	19	19	18	18	17	17
8.9	55	25	24	24	23	22	21	21	20	19	19	18	18	17	17
8.11	56	26	25	24	23	22	22	21	21	20	19	19	18	18	17
9	57	26	25	25	24	23	22	21	21	20	20	19	19	18	18
9.2	58	27	26	25	24	23	23	22	21	21	20	19	19	18	18
9.4	59	27	26	26	25	24	23	22	22	21	20	20	19	19	18
9.6	60	28	27	26	25	24	23	23	22	21	21	20	20	19	19
9.9	61	28	27	26	25	24	24	23	22	22	21	20	20	19	19
9.11	62	29	28	27	26	25	24	23	23	22	21	21	20	20	19
9.13	63	29	28	27	26	25	25	24	23	22	22	21	21	20	19
10.1	64	30	28	28	27	26	25	24	24	23	22	21	21	20	20
10.3	65	30	29	28	27	26	25	24	24	23	22	22	21	21	20
10.6	66	31	29	29	27	26	26	25	24	23	23	22	22	21	20
10.8	67	31	30	29	28	27	26	25	25	24	23	22	22	21	21
10.10	68	31	30	29	28	27	27	26	25	24	24	23	22	21	21
10.12	69	32	31	30	29	28	27	26	25	24	24	23	23	22	21
11	70	32	31	30	29	28	27	26	26	25	24	23	23	22	22
11.3	71	33	32	31	30	28	28	27	26	25	25	24	23	22	22
11.5	72	33	32	31	30	29	28	27	26	26	25	24	24	23	22
11.7	73	34	32	32	30	29	29	27	27	26	25	24	24	23	23
11.9	74	34	33	32	31	30	29	28	27	26	26	25	24	23	23
11.11	75	35	33	32	31	30	29	28	28	27	26	25	24	24	23
12	76	35	34	33	32	30	29	28	28	27	26	25	25	24	23
12.2	77	36	34	33	32	31	30	29	28	27	27	26	25	24	24
12.4	78	36	35	34	32	31	30	29	29	28	27	26	25	25	24
12.6	79	37	35	34	33	32	31	30	29	28	27	26	26	25	24
12.8	80	37	36	35	33	32	31	30	29	28	28	27	26	25	25
12.11	81	37	36	35	34	32	32	30	30	29	28	27	26	26	25
12.13	82	38	36	35	34	33	32	31	30	29	28	27	27	26	25
13.1	83	38	37	36	35	33	32	31	30	29	29	28	27	26	26
13.3	84	39	37	36	35	34	33	32	31	30	29	28	27	27	26
13.5	85	39	38	37	35	34	33	32	31	30	29	28	28	27	26
13.8	86	40	38	37	36	34	34	32	32	30	30	29	28	27	27
13.10	87	40	39	38	36	35	34	33	32	31	30	29	28	27	27
	cms	147	150	152	155	158	160	163	165	168	170	173	175	178	180
	ft	4.10	4.11	5.0	5.1	5.2	5.3	5.4	5.5	5.6	5.7	5.8	5.9	5.10	5.11

Imperial measures given are only approximates

BMI = kg/m^2

Body Mass Index Chart

What is Underweight?

Anything under a BMI of 20 is considered underweight and could make it difficult for you to conceive. This is one of nature's protective mechanisms. The theory is that if we do not have enough fat stores our bodies think we are starving. Since it is not appropriate to become pregnant when food is short, ovulation or menstruation stop. (This is why women of the bushmen tribes only ovulate at a certain time of year when food is plentiful.[80]) When our weight gets back to normal (because we have stopped dieting and/or reduced the amount of exercise we take) we start ovulating and menstruating again. Our bodies assume that food is now plentiful and we become fertile again.

And even short-term dieting can have an effect. For example, healthy women who were put on a diet of 1,000 calories a day for just six weeks showed hormonal disruption in that short time. Progesterone, the important hormone which maintains pregnancy, dropped significantly and so did their oestrogen levels.[81]

The good news is that getting back to the right weight really does boost your fertility. One study showed that nearly three-quarters of women with unexplained infertility managed to conceive naturally once they stopped dieting and returned to a normal weight.[82]

If you get your weight back up to normal quickly it is still advisable to wait at least four months before trying to conceive. You will almost certainly have some vitamin and mineral deficiencies because you have been restricting your food intake. The four-month wait before getting pregnant is vital because otherwise, if you have been undernourished, you are more likely to have a low birthweight baby.

As we have seen, the current popularity of no-fat or low-fat foods and diets has some serious implications for fertility. Dieting in this way may deprive you of the nutrients that are essential for the proper functioning of your reproductive system. Just how serious an effect this can have was demonstrated by one study which showed that only 27 per cent of the women on a fat-restricted diet were actually ovulating.[83]

To improve your fertility you should aim for a BMI within the normal range of 20–25, the optimum being 24.[84]

Food should be eaten regularly and you should never skip meals. Apart from ensuring that you are well-nourished, regular meals are important to maintain your hormonal balance (see page 36).

What is Overweight?

A BMI of over 25 is considered overweight and it can reduce your fertility. However, just losing a small amount of weight, say 10 per cent, can be enough to improve your hormone profiles, make your periods more regular, stimulate ovulation and increase your chances of pregnancy.[85]

In fact it has been suggested that changing a woman's diet should be the first move if she is overweight and failing to conceive.[86] And research shows that even women with normal ovaries gain positive improvements in their hormone balance as they lose weight.[86]

However, once you are pregnant, dieting is positively harmful. This is because, when you diet, your body gets rid of toxins and waste products. This is usually a good thing but if you are pregnant then the toxins can go straight into the developing baby.

For this reason, you must aim to lose any excess weight *before* you get pregnant. If you are already pregnant, then it is fine to change the quality of your food (by buying healthier foods such as organic vegetables, changing to organic free-range eggs, eliminating sugar, etc) but you still need to eat a good variety of food and not skip meals.

Hormones and Blood Sugar

The key to the link between excess weight and reduced fertility lies in the way your blood sugar levels (which are controlled by your diet and eating habits) affect your hormonal cycle. If the first is not in balance, then your hormones (which control your fertility) may not work properly either.

This link was recognised by Dr Katharine Dalton, a pioneer in the treatment of pre-menstrual syndrome (PMS), who discovered that her patients' PMS symptoms were relieved by eating regularly. The 'little and often' approach to eating prevents the blood sugar levels from dropping excessively and stops adrenalin from being released. What Dr Dalton discovered was that this adrenalin blocked the utilisation (or uptake) of progesterone in the second half of the menstrual cycle. This problem, ultimately due to poor eating habits, was causing the symptoms of PMS. The answer was to stabilise blood sugar levels by getting patients to eat properly and stop the adrenaline interfering with the progesterone.

Interestingly, when women with PMS are tested, their blood hormone levels, including progesterone, are no different from those of women without PMS. The difference is not that PMS sufferers have low progesterone levels but that, because of their low blood sugar levels (hypoglycaemia), their bodies cannot use the progesterone they have.

This discovery has huge implications for fertility and miscarriage problems. If progesterone is blocked in this way it reduces the chances of maintaining a pregnancy, since (as we saw on page 39), this hormone is needed to maintain the womb lining at the very start of a pregnancy. Many women who think they are infertile may therefore actually get pregnant without knowing but lose the embryo early on because their bodies cannot use the progesterone they have. In such cases they may believe they are just having a normal period.

There is also a clear and well-established link between blood sugar balance problems such as diabetes, poor eating habits and excess weight. If you are not eating properly your blood sugar levels can zoom up and down chaotically. Not only can this have the hormonal effect observed by Dr Dalton but it may also spark off the sugar cravings, food obsessions and bingeing habits that make us eat even more of the wrong food and put on even more weight. So it is a vicious circle.

Why Does Your Blood Sugar Level Rise and Fall?

After a meal, glucose produced by the breakdown of food (digestion) is absorbed through the wall of the intestine into the bloodstream. At this point, there is, quite naturally, a high level of glucose in the blood. Your body takes what it immediately needs for energy and then produces insulin from the pancreas in an attempt to reduce the excess. Glucose that is not used immediately for energy is changed into glycogen and stored in the liver and muscles to be used later. It's this finely tuned system that usually keeps the glucose level in your blood at a healthy well-balanced norm.

To maintain this balance, your body works in a similar way to the thermostat on a central heating system. Just as the thermostat clicks into action as temperatures rise or fall, so your natural 'thermostat' clicks into action as glucose levels rise and fall. When your 'thermostat' recognises that there is too much or too little, your body takes action:

• When the glucose level falls too low adrenalin is released by the adrenal glands and glucagon is produced by the pancreas. Glucagon works in the opposite way to insulin and increases blood glucose by encouraging the liver to turn some of its glycogen stores into glucose to give us quick energy.

- If the blood glucose level stays low for a period of time, hypoglycaemia – low blood sugar – can occur. Symptoms include irritability, aggressive outbursts, palpitations, forgetfulness, lack of sex drive, crying spells, dizziness, fears and anxiety, confusion, inability to concentrate, fatigue, insomnia, headaches, muscle cramps, excessive sweating and excessive thirst.
- Alternatively, when the glucose level rises too high, insulin is produced by the pancreas to lower it. If the blood sugar level remains too high, this causes the symptoms of hyperglycaemia – high blood sugar level. The extreme form of this is diabetes. With this condition, insulin is supplied from outside the body by injection to bring the level down. The greater your weight, the higher your risk of developing diabetes. Obese people have a 77 times higher chance of developing it.

During a normal day, the amount by which your blood sugar level rises and falls depends on two main factors: what and when you eat or drink.

What You Eat or Drink

When you eat any food in a refined form you digest it very fast. Refined foods are no longer in their 'whole' state and have been stripped of their natural goodness by various manufacturing processes. Two of the most widely used refined foods are sugar and white flour.

If digestion is too fast then glucose enters the bloodstream too rapidly. This also happens when you eat any food or drink that gives a stimulant effect, like tea, coffee or chocolate. This sharp, fast rise in blood glucose, which makes you feel good temporarily, is always followed by a rapid drop.

The initial stimulating 'high' quickly passes, and you plummet down to a 'low' in which you feel tired and drained. So what do you need? Another stimulant, like a bar of chocolate or a cup of coffee (or both!), to give you another boost.

This second boost causes your blood sugar level to go up rapidly again and the vicious cycle is repeated. All this causes an up-and-down, roller-coaster of blood sugar swings, which in turn causes a roller-coaster of eating patterns and cravings for sweet foods and drinks which lead to weight gain.

Over time, this constant over-stimulation exhausts the pancreas. Then, instead of too much insulin, it produces too little. And too much glucose stays in the blood, causing the symptoms of high blood sugar levels.

When You Eat or Drink

If there is a long gap between meals your blood glucose will drop to quite a low level, leaving you feeling the need for a quick boost (say a cup of tea and a biscuit). At the same time, your adrenal glands will make your liver produce more glucose. The combination of these two causes high levels of glucose in your blood, which again calls on the pancreas to over-produce insulin in order to reduce your glucose levels. The roller-coaster ride starts all over again and your adrenal glands become even more exhausted.

The answer to this particular problem is simple. Develop a 'grazing' mentality – eating little and often is best.

The Effects of Adrenalin

If your blood sugar levels are frequently low and your system is regularly being asked to pump out adrenaline your health and fertility will suffer. Adrenalin is the hormone most of us associate with stress. It is the hormone that is released for 'fight or flight' and its effect is very powerful. The heart speeds up and the arteries tighten to raise blood pressure. (That's what causes your heart to pound when you are frightened.) Your liver immediately releases emergency stores of glucose into your bloodstream to give you instant energy to fight or run. And your digestion stops, because it is not necessary for immediate survival so your body needn't waste time and energy on it. The clotting ability of your blood is also increased in case of injury. This all means that you have been made ready to run faster, fight back and generally react more quickly than normal.

Unfortunately, when your blood sugar level drops during the day or night, adrenaline is released automatically and your body experiences all the above sensations – except that there is no outside stress to respond to. These surges of adrenalin can contribute to heart disease by increasing the risk of blood clotting and high blood pressure, and they can also cause extreme fluctuations of sugar levels in your blood due to the sudden release of glucose.

Apart from these negative effects on your general health, the release of adrenalin will block your body's ability to utilise progesterone, which is vital in maintaining a pregnancy.

How Can You Balance Your Blood Sugar?

To balance your blood sugar, you need to follow three golden rules:

1. Eat complex carbohydrates regularly.
2. Avoid refined foods, especially sugar.
3. Reduce foods and drinks that are stimulants.

1. Eat Complex Carbohydrates Regularly

You need to eat foods that give a slow rise in blood sugar and keep a constant level for about three hours. Then you need to eat again, to prevent the level from dropping. Spacing food at three-hourly intervals in this way maintains a good balance.

And the best foods for this are complex carbohydrates (see page 50). They give a slow release of energy because it takes time for the digestive tract to break them down into simpler substances that the body can use.

To help maintain a steady blood sugar level, aim to eat complex carbohydrates as part of your main meals and also regularly during the day. You do not necessarily need to eat large amounts. Sometimes just an oatcake between meals can be enough to keep eating urges at bay.

If you find the symptoms associated with low blood sugar level are greatest first thing in the morning or you wake during the night, heart pounding, and cannot get back to sleep, then it is very likely that your blood sugar level has dropped overnight and adrenalin has been released. Eating a small, starchy snack, like an oatcake, one hour before going to bed and, if possible, one hour after getting up, will help to alleviate these symptoms.

2. Avoid Refined Foods, Especially Sugar

Simple carbohydrates, with the exception of fruit, are all refined foods and should be avoided. Although fruit contains fructose (fruit sugar), which is a simple sugar, the fibre content of the fruit is a complex carbohydrate which slows the digestion rate. So fructose is acceptable when taken in the whole fruit, like an apple, but not when used in the refined form of powdered white fructose bought in boxes.

Pure fruit juice can also cause a rapid change in blood sugar level because it is not buffered by the fibre that is normally present in the fruit. It is therefore better to dilute fruit juice in water to make it less concentrated.

Sugar seems to be everywhere, even in unexpected places. And, by the way, the 'brown-is-best rule' doesn't apply to sugar. All colours do the same damage to your blood sugar balance!

A can of cola may contain up to eight teaspoons of sugar, as may a pot of fruit yogurt. Most of the convenience foods and drinks we buy are laden with it. Sugar is also in savoury foods, such as baked beans and mayonnaise. Did you know that tomato ketchup has just 8 per cent less sugar, weight for weight, than ice cream, and that the cream substitute used for coffee is 65 per cent sugar (compared to 51 per cent for a chocolate bar)?

Indeed, sugar is added to practically everything, as it is an inexpensive bulking agent. Even some toothpastes contain sugar but, as toothpaste is not a food, sugar does not have to be included on the ingredients list.

Sugar is just 'empty' calories. This means that it contains no nutritional value so you can happily cut it out and lose nothing but weight. You may be tempted to replace sugar with artificial sweeteners – don't. You are simply substituting an alien chemical which your body then has to deal with, giving it extra work to do. Nobody really knows what havoc these chemicals may cause when introduced into our own bodies' delicately balanced biochemistry.

If a food or drink is described as 'low sugar' or 'diet' it will usually contain an artificial chemical sweetener such as saccharin or aspartame. They are also found in some non-diet crisps, ice lollies, sauces, pot noodles and some over-the-counter medicines so it's worth checking labels carefully.

3. Reduce Foods and Drinks That are Stimulants

Sugar, smoking and caffeine in tea, coffee, chocolate and caffeinated soft drinks, are all stimulants and cause a fast rise in blood sugar level, followed by a quick drop. Avoid them whenever possible. Or, even better, cut them out of your diet completely. Replace with herbal teas and grain coffee, spring water and diluted pure fruit juices.

Summary

Do:

- Eat plenty of unrefined complex carbohydrates, including wholewheat bread, wholemeal pasta, potatoes, brown rice, millet, oats and rye.
- Eat fruit and drink diluted pure fruit juice.
- Always eat breakfast – porridge oats are good.
- Eat small, frequent meals no more than three hours apart.
- Reduce, and preferably avoid, stimulants including tea, coffee, chocolate, smoking and canned drinks that contain caffeine.

Don't:

- Eat refined carbohydrates. Avoid 'white' in general. Remember that white flour is in many foods, like cakes, biscuits, pastries and white bread.
- Eat sugar or foods containing it, including chocolate, sweets, biscuits, pastries and soft drinks.
- Replace coffee with decaffeinated coffee (as it contains two other stimulants, even when the caffeine is removed).
- Eat convenience foods, as they are likely to contain refined carbohydrates, sugar and high levels of fat and salt.

Shopping for Healthy Food

The key is to buy food in its most natural state. As a general rule, avoid foods that have had chemicals added (either to replace something natural, as with artificial sweeteners) or to prolong shelf-life.

Remember that you are aiming to avoid chemicals that could compromise your fertility. You also want to optimise your health by eating as naturally as possible, in order to increase your chances of getting pregnant.

The first step is to get into the habit of reading labels carefully.

Reading Labels

Although most of us lead busy lives, and tend to do our shopping as quickly as possible, it's worth investing some time in looking at labels on foods and drinks before you buy them. Once you are familiar with the best brands to buy, shopping for the healthiest foods becomes relatively easy.

Firstly, it is best to avoid ingredients which sound like something from a chemistry lesson, especially products containing E numbers. Some are fine to eat, as they are naturally derived, but the vast majority are not and have known side-effects. Without carrying a reference book with us all the time we cannot know which ones are which. Usually food manufacturers make it clear if the additive in question is a natural one because it is a good selling point. However, if in doubt, avoid it altogether.

Also check the label for artificial sweeteners (such as saccharin and aspartame) and, where possible, avoid them. They are chemicals too and the safety of many of them is in doubt.

Generally, the longer the ingredients list, the more suspicious you should be about the product.

Manufacturers argue that additives, preservatives and flavourings are used in such small quantities that they have no adverse effect. However, if you take into account the cumulative effect of these additives in all the different products you eat each day, the quantities soon mount up. Nobody knows what the combined effect of this chemical cocktail might be or how it could affect fertility and a developing baby.

These days it's more or less impossible for most people to make sure that every single thing they eat is chemical-free, especially if their lifestyle means they need to eat snacks or meals away from home. But, without getting unduly anxious about it, you need to eat as naturally and healthily as possible. For example, as you will undoubtedly need to buy convenience or packaged food from time to time, try to find the best brand you can by going for the shortest, most chemical-free ingredients list.

HEALTHY COOKING TIPS

- With organic carrots and potatoes, you only need to scrub the skins. Do not peel them, as many of the nutrients are concentrated just under the skin.
- To avoid nutrient loss, lightly cook vegetables in a little water or steam them.
- Avoid frying where possible. Try grilling or baking instead.
- Choose cookware with care. Avoid all aluminium cookware, as this is a heavy toxic metal that can enter food through the cooking process. The same applies to aluminium foil and cases. Avoid any coated cookware, such as non-stick, which is thought to be carcinogenic. The best cookware materials are cast iron, enamel, glass and stainless steel.

Making the Right Choices

Variety is the key to enjoying your food and eating for health, fertility and pregnancy. You need to choose your food carefully, because healthy food means healthy babies. Most supermarkets now stock quite a lot of organic produce. But you can also try shopping at healthfood shops and organic farm shops, some of which offer a mail order service.

Fruit and Vegetables

Buying organic produce will enable you to avoid pesticides, DDT and Kepone. These contain xenoestrogens which are oestrogen-like compounds that can upset the delicate male and female hormone balance (see page 36). Although DDT is banned in the UK, it is still used in some developing countries and can therefore enter our food chain through imported produce. Organic food also contains more of the valuable nutrients which are essential for fertility. You should include plenty of organic fresh fruit and vegetables in your diet. Fruit is very versatile and can be enjoyed at any time of the day.

Dried fruits make a nice change, but you should avoid any that contain the preserving agent sulphur dioxide which is also used as a bleaching agent in flour. Sulphur dioxide occurs naturally but is produced chemically for commercial use. It is suspected of being a factor in genetic mutations and also of irritating the alimentary canal.

Supermarket dried fruits, such as mixed fruit, raisins and sultanas, often have mineral oil added to them to give them a shiny appearance and keep them separate. Try to avoid this kind of oil, as it can interfere with your absorption of calcium and phosphorus. As it passes through your body, mineral oil can pick up and excrete the oil-soluble vitamins (A, D, E and K) which you really want to retain.

Grains

If you only have a limited amount to spend on organic produce, then buy organic grains if nothing else. This is because grains are very small and can absorb more pesticides than other foods.

Breakfast Cereals

Shredded Wheat and Puffed Wheat (and supermarket own brands of these) are sugar-free. There are also a number of good no-added sugar mueslis and cereals available from healthfood shops and supermarkets now.

Muesli contains raw flakes of various grains and should be soaked for a minimum of ten minutes before eating, but soaking overnight is definitely best. Soaking enables the phytates (which can block the uptake of minerals from food) to be broken down properly.

Breads

Organic wholemeal bread is best and healthfood shops and supermarkets stock some good ones such as Shipton Mill. Some breads contain either sugar or dextrose and/or flour improvers, so read the labels carefully. If the flour improver is ascorbic acid, that's OK as it is a form of vitamin C. Wholemeal pitta bread makes a nice change but do check the label for undesirable ingredients.

Flavourings

Avoid over-processed, commercially-produced flavourings. Instead, choose from ginger, garlic, fresh and dried herbs, lemon juice, sea salt, Lo-salt, miso (soya bean paste), mustard (check for added sugar, chemicals, etc), and arrowroot for thickening to make gravies and sauces.

Soya sauce is good on rice, in salad dressings and sauces, as well as Chinese stir-fries. Choose organic where possible and avoid any makes which contain monosodium glutamate. There are also a number of ready-made salad dressings with no sugar or chemicals, but do check the labels.

Sweeteners

It is better to rely on the natural sweetness in foods rather than using artificial sweeteners. For example, if you are making cakes, try carrot and raisin or banana cake. However, if you do want to add a sweetener, use maple syrup, concentrated apple juice, barley malt, date syrup and honey.

When buying honey, avoid those which are 'blended' or the 'produce of more than one country', as they are often heated to temperatures as high as 71°C (160°F) which destroys their goodness. With maple syrup, if the label says 'flavoured' beware: if it is not the real thing it could contain sugar and chemical flavouring.

Beans/Pulses

Beans make a good base for many healthy dishes, especially if you are trying to stay off meat to improve your fertility. They are great added to salads, soups and casseroles, and you'll find them a useful and economical addition to your culinary repertoire.

Most beans (not lentils) need to be soaked, some overnight, before cooking. Alternatively, you can buy organic beans in tins from most supermarkets which have a little salt added to them but no sugar.

Houmous, which is made from chickpeas, can be bought ready-made from most supermarkets and is a good source of protein and essential fatty acids.

Meat

Meat is high in saturated fat so you should try to cut down on it. Of all meat, poultry is the healthiest choice and several supermarkets now sell organic, free-range or corn-fed birds, all of which are preferable to the usual mass-produced birds. However, apart from saturated fat, meat also contains growth hormones, antibiotics and other chemicals given to many animals reared for human consumption.

In addition to its adverse effects on fertility, these is also a possible link between the consumption of red meat and bowel cancer. The Government has therefore suggested that our intake of red meat should be less than 90g (3.2oz) a day.

Fish

Fish has low saturated fat levels and is very nutritious. It's best to grill or poach fish, rather than fry it. Oily fish is particularly good, as it contains high levels of essential fatty acids, so you can enjoy mackerel, tuna, salmon (eat the bones), sardines and anchovies. Fresh is best but frozen or tinned are acceptable.

Eggs

Buy organic free-range eggs. You want organic as well as free-range. 'Free-range' only implies that the hens, unlike their battery cousins, have been given a certain amount of freedom but they can still be fed on 'junk'.

Soya

Soya is a very versatile, natural vegetable protein which can make a useful alternative to cow's milk if you are animal milk intolerant or find that it causes skin problems or sinus trouble. Buy organic to make sure it is not genetically modified and make sure the milk is sugar-free. Soya milk can be used in cooking in the same way as you would use cow's milk and you will find you then cannot taste the difference between the two.

Tofu which is soya bean curd can be used in stir-fries, soups and also desserts and again buy organic to make sure it is GM free. It is available in most supermarkets and healthfood shops. Avoid TVP (textured vegetable protein) because of the amount of processing needed to make it into a meat substitute.

Dairy Produce

Buy organic dairy produce, available from most supermarkets, to avoid the harmful effects of growth hormones, antibiotics and chemicals that may have been absorbed from the animal's foodstuffs. If you have a milk allergy or intolerance, try sheep's or goat's milk or a non-animal drink like soya milk or rice milk. Buy live yogurt containing the culture *Lactobacillus acidophilus* – organic if possible.

Oil/Fat

Use butter (organic if possible) and unhydrogenated margarines (available from healthfood shops). Look for cold-pressed, unrefined vegetable oils like sesame, sunflower and safflower, and use extra-virgin olive oil for light cooking.

Hot Drinks

As a substitute for coffee, try Caro and Caro Extra, Bambu or Yannoh which are grain 'coffees' and contain various combinations of ingredients like barley, rye, chicory and acorns. Good alternatives to tea include herb teas, fruit teas, Rooibos (caffeine-free South African tea), decaffeinated tea, or Japanese bancha (twig) tea.

Cold Drinks

Use real unsweetened fruit juice. Watch out for cartons or bottles with 'fruit drink' on the label because this means that something else has been added. A recent analysis of fruit drinks showed that many contained only 5 per cent fruit, while the rest was made up with water, sugar and additives.

Also be cautious of the flavoured spring waters. They appear healthy enough but many contain sugar.

Water is the simplest and most natural drink of all. Our bodies are made up of approximately 70 per cent water which is essential for every bodily process. We can survive without food for about five weeks but we can't go without water for longer than five days.

Try to drink around six glasses of water a day. Use these glasses of water to replace other less healthy drinks you might normally choose. For instance, you could start the day with a cup of hot water and a slice of lemon, a wonderfully refreshing drink and excellent for the liver.

TAP OR BOTTLED WATER?

Unfortunately your tap water may be contaminated with any number of impurities. Arsenic, copper and lead can all occur naturally and they sometimes leach into the water from the pipes. Similarly, other substances, such as pesticides and fertilisers, can leach into the water from the ground.

   I would therefore suggest that you get a filter (either a jug filter or one plumbed in under the sink) and use water from that for cooking vegetables, making hot drinks, etc. A filter cannot eliminate every impurity, but it is a start. You may prefer bottled water for drinking, so here is a short buyers' guide:

• **Spring water** may have been taken from one or more underground sources and have undergone a range of treatments (such as filtration and blending).

• **Natural mineral water** is bottled in its natural state (without treatment). It has to come from an officially registered source, conform to purity standards, and carry details of its source and mineral analysis on the label.

• **Naturally sparkling water** must come from its underground source with enough natural carbon dioxide to make it bubbly.

• **Sparkling (carbonated) water** has carbon dioxide added to it during bottling (as with ordinary fizzy drinks).

Convenience Foods

Most pre-packaged convenience foods contain high levels of additives and preservatives so they are best avoided. However, even with the best will in the world, I know this is not always possible. So, when you do feel you have to buy convenience foods, check the labels carefully, go for organic options where available, and keep your consumption of such foods to a minimum.

CHAPTER 8

Giving Up Alcohol, Smoking and Drugs

I have seen many couples who based their social life around drinking and smoking because they had failed to start a family. Yet these may well have been the very factors that were stopping them conceiving. Those of them who followed the recommendations in this chapter and successfully conceived say that, although the changes seemed daunting at the time, they now seem only a small sacrifice.

Men are often reluctant to eliminate alcohol but I usually remind the male partner that he only has to give up drinking until the woman gets pregnant. It's us women who have to stay off it for the whole nine months (see Chapter 24).

If you still need convincing, it may help to look at a brief sample of recent research on the damage alcohol and smoking do to fertility and the unborn child.

Alcohol

Alcohol is a mutagen, which means it is a substance that can cause mutations.

Studies have shown that giving male mice alcohol damaged their sperm and increased the number of still-born or miscarried offspring by three times. And female rats given alcohol before ovulation had lower fertility and an increased number of dead and deformed offspring. The most extreme effect of alcohol is demonstrated by the fact that 80 per cent of chronic alcoholic men are sterile and alcohol is a common cause of impotence.[88]

Your partner should wait at least four months to clear his reproductive system from the effects of alcohol before you try to conceive. This is because sperm take about that long to mature. Sperm that mature while alcohol is still in the system may be less healthy and effective.[89]

The other reason to give up drinking well in advance of conception is that when you get pregnant it will be at least two weeks before you know it. Toxins from drinking and smoking alcohol are at their most dangerous during the first few weeks of pregnancy because embryo cell division is at its highest then.

Smoking

Couples who smoke have high levels of cadmium, a heavy toxic metal that can stop the utilisation of zinc needed for both male and female fertility. Cadmium will not leave the body just because you or your partner stop smoking. It needs to be actively tackled by supplementing your diet with antioxidant supplements (see Chapter 10). Even if you give up smoking the cadmium already in your body can concentrate in the placenta once you get pregnant.[90] So it's important to be tested for heavy toxic metals (see Chapter 12) and make sure that your levels are back to normal before you try to conceive.

What if your partner smokes? Research has shown that chemicals in tobacco smoke can damage the DNA in sperm and deplete the amount of vitamin E, which works as an antioxidant, protecting the sperm. But there is a bigger potential problem resulting from your partner smoking. Dramatic findings from an Oxford Survey on Childhood Cancers, published in 1997 in the *British Journal of Cancer*,[91] found that men who smoke when their partner doesn't run a higher risk of fathering children who develop cancer. One in seven childhood cancers, including leukaemia and brain tumours, could be due to the father's smoking habits. Just 1–9 cigarettes per day increased the risk by 3 per cent, 10–20 by 31 per cent and 20 or more cigarettes by 42 per cent. The study concluded that the man risks damaging his sperm more, the more he smokes.

So alcohol and smoking clearly affect fertility for both men and women. If you are really serious about getting pregnant they therefore have to be eliminated for at least four months to give you the best possible chance. I cannot say 'a little bit won't harm' because it certainly can if it is at a vital stage of egg or sperm development.

How to Stop Smoking

Acupuncture can be extremely helpful to get over the withdrawal symptoms when you give up smoking, and I have seen many couples who have used hypnotherapy successfully. I have listed the Quitline telephone number under Useful Addresses (see page 228).

You should not use nicotine patches, nicotine gum or any other anti-smoking aids of this kind once you have started the Four-Month Preconception Plan (see Section 6).

Case History

Ann was 30 when she came to see me in summer 1997 after suffering three miscarriages in quick succession. Her mother had had difficulties as well – she had lost one baby at four months old, and had had three miscarriages. She had told Ann that as a result she had been 'pumped full of hormones' while she was expecting her, to stop her miscarrying. Ann worked long and stressful hours as a stockbroker and felt exhausted. Her partner also worked long and stressful hours and smoked 20 cigarettes a day with 5 units of alcohol each weekday and 10 each day at the weekend. Ann drank every day but less than her partner. We discussed the effects of all these factors on the risk of miscarriage. They were tested for genito-urinary infections but these were negative.

Their mineral results were very interesting. Her partner had extremely low levels of zinc and unacceptable levels of cadmium, the toxic poison present in tobacco smoke. Cadmium, like alcohol, can be teratogenic which means that it can cause abnormalities in the foetus. The autopsy on the last miscarriage had shown chromosomal abnormalities but both Ann and her partner were tested for genetic problems and both were fine. So the abnormality was not inherited from the parents but was caused by something happening to the developing cells around conception. Ann's tests also showed that she was low in zinc and manganese.

I explained to them that their best chance of preventing another miscarriage was to stop drinking, which they did, and Ann's partner also stopped smoking. They also made other changes, by looking at their diet and lifestyle, and waited four months until they were both back to optimum health before trying again. Ann then became pregnant and had a healthy baby boy. She wrote to me later, saying that they were convinced that the preconception plan I suggested they followed, as outlined in this book, not only helped them have the baby and avoid another miscarriage but that people had commented on how healthy and contented he is.

Eliminating Drugs

If you or your partner are addicted to any drugs, it is important that you seek professional help by talking to your doctor. He or she can then refer you to a specialist to help overcome the addiction and to allow time for the drugs to be cleared out of your bodies before conception.

If your doctor has prescribed medication for either you or your partner then ask him or her to check whether the drug has any side-effects which could affect fertility. If the drug is essential then ask if there is another type which does not have those side-effects. Also ask if the medication is absolutely essential and if it is not, you may be able to stop taking it.

CHAPTER 9

Reducing Your Stress Levels

Stress can affect both male and female fertility, and not conceiving can in itself become a cause of stress. Many women with fertility problems say that their whole life seems to revolve round their monthly cycle – hoping their period will not come, and, when it does, feeling devastated, and that yet another month has been 'wasted'. The couple's relationship may be put under severe strain during the rounds of investigations and IVF treatments. For example, one woman who came to see me, after previous unsuccessful IVF treatments, became pregnant naturally. But then her husband left her, saying he never wanted a baby anyway. He had gone with her for numerous IVF treatments but none of this had been spoken about. In such cases counselling may well be helpful (see Useful Addresses).

If stress is a factor for you, then it is also worth learning some form of relaxation, stress management technique or meditation. Hypnotherapy can also be helpful, in that it can work on the subconscious to address emotional blockages. (For information on all these, see Useful Addresses.)

When you are desperate to conceive, lovemaking can lose its spontaneity as there is the feeling that intercourse must happen on certain days of the month and those days mustn't be missed. However, research has shown that the more enjoyable the lovemaking (and especially if the woman has an orgasm), the more likely she is to retain more active sperm. The contractions caused by the orgasm draw in more sperm and it is thought that her arousal may make the vagina less acidic, increasing the chances of the sperm surviving longer. I think the message is: enjoy yourselves!

Coping with Sleep Problems

If you take tranquillisers or sleeping pills, talk to your doctor about gradually coming off them and finding an alternative. Herbs can be very helpful. Valerian is a wonderful herb for helping with insomnia and it is classed as a sedative in herbal medicine. Passionflower (or passiflora) is another good herb for helping you sleep and can be used together with valerian for maximum effect. A cup of hot camomile tea before bed can also be effective.

Aromatherapy oils, such as bergamot, lavender and camomile, can be added to a relaxing warm bath just before going to bed.

Magnesium, known as 'nature's tranquilliser', is a good mineral to use when weaning yourself off conventional medication. One dose of magnesium (100mg) can be taken about an hour before you go to bed.

CHAPTER 10

Taking Nutritional Supplements

There is now a great deal of scientific knowledge about the use of nutritional supplements and their beneficial effects on both male and female fertility. As you will see, these supplements can be very effective in rebalancing your hormones, as well as improving your and your partner's overall health – so vital for successful conception.

Unfortunately, you would not normally hear about the value of supplements from your doctor, yet the suggestions made in this book are backed up by medical and scientific evidence, and there are good reasons for following them.

Firstly, you need to supplement your diet because, with all the good intentions in the world, it is hard nowadays to get all the nutrients you need just from the food you eat. For instance, our daily intake of selenium (34mcg) is now only half the amount it was 25 years ago. And this amount is half the minimum 75mcg a day recommended for men and 60mcg recommended for women. This is because, even if you eat the 'right' food, modern agricultural and production processes remove much of its goodness.

The aim of this book is to increase your and your partner's fertility over a four-month period. To ensure that you take in the right amount of nutrients in that short space of time, you really have to take supplements. For optimum nutrition, healthy fertility and successful conception, each of the following nutrients is essential in your diet.

Folic Acid

Folic acid deficiency is the most common vitamin deficiency in the world,[92] partly because the body cannot store large amounts of folic acid. It really only has sufficient for one to two months so it is essential to supplement.

Of course, we now know that folic acid can prevent spina bifida and it is essential that it is in good supply before and during pregnancy. But that is not all.

Folic acid is just one of a number of B vitamins. To successfully produce the genetic materials DNA and RNA, you must have enough folic acid, together with vitamin B12. This co-dependency is common between nutrients and, because of such interactions, it is naive to think that supplementing with folic acid alone before pregnancy, as suggested by the medical profession, is enough.

You have to remember that doctors are not generally trained in nutrition. (They receive only a few lectures on the subject while they are studying if they are lucky.) By giving advice in isolation and without the necessary nutritional training, other complications can arise. For example, since folic acid and vitamin B12 are inextricably linked, it is possible to mask a B12 deficiency (pernicious anaemia), for instance, by giving folic acid alone.[93]

A US study found that women taking a multivitamin before conception had fewer babies with a cleft lip. The immediate assumption was that it was probably the folic acid that was making the difference. But, since all the other vitamins were also being taken, it could have been any one of them that had the positive benefit. More likely, it was the combination of all the nutrients.[94]

Recent research into heart disease suggests that folic acid and vitamin B12 might be beneficial in controlling an amino acid called homocysteine, found in the blood, that causes damage to the lining of blood vessels. Since high levels of homocysteine are also found in women who have miscarriages, it surely follows that folic acid and vitamin B12 might be helpful to these women too.[95]

When trying to get pregnant, you should also be aware that folic acid deficiency is common in people with chronic diarrhoea or malabsorptive states such as coeliac disease and Crohn's disease. Alcohol causes the body to excrete folic acid, and certain drugs, such as those for epilepsy and oral contraceptives, can cause a folic acid deficiency. So, if you fall into any of the above categories, make sure you supplement with folic acid before trying to get pregnant.[96]

You should take 400mcg a day. (You also need to take vitamin B12 – see page 86)

Zinc

Zinc is the most widely studied nutrient in terms of fertility for both men and women. It is an essential component of genetic material, and a zinc deficiency can cause chromosome changes in either the man or the woman, leading to reduced fertility and an increased risk of miscarriages.

Zinc is necessary for the body to attract and hold the reproductive hormones, oestrogen and progesterone.[97]

Zinc also plays a vital role in cell division so it is especially important that adequate levels are available at the time of conception. When couples go for IVF treatment, and the egg has been fertilised, the doctors have to wait until it divides sufficiently before it is put back in the woman. If the cell division is inadequate then that fertilised egg will not be used. This same cell division takes place during natural conception and it also requires good levels of zinc. If levels are not optimum, then it not only makes it difficult to conceive but there are also risks of having a baby with low birthweight, malformations or poor development of the brain and nervous system.[98]

Zinc deficiency can block the absorption of folic acid so having a deficiency of one nutrient can lead to deficiencies in other nutrients. This is why getting a good intake of a number of nutrients is so important.[99]

Zinc is also vital for your partner because it is crucial for the proper development of sperm.[100] We know this because when young animals are fed a zinc-deficient diet they can produce abnormal sperm.[101] For example, 60 day-old mice were found to be sterile after only three weeks of being fed a zinc-deficient diet.[102]

Studies carried out in the 1980s showed that zinc deficiency in men causes a temporary but reversible reduction in sperm count and a reduced testosterone level.[103] And this reduction in testosterone level has since been confirmed by other studies.[104]

Giving zinc to men with low testosterone levels raises the hormone to a more normal level and increases the sperm count. In one study some men had an increase of 150 per cent in their sperm count, and in nine cases out of 22 their partners conceived while they were taking the zinc.[105]

Simply comparing men with low sperm counts to men with normal sperm counts has shown that serum (blood) zinc levels and seminal zinc levels are significantly lower in infertile men.[106]

With each ejaculation, men lose up to 9 per cent of their daily zinc intake.[107] So it is crucial that your partner keeps up a good daily intake of zinc.

Clearly, zinc should be taken as a supplement if there is any problem with sperm count or quality. You and your partner should also include sources of zinc, such as oats, rye, wholewheat, almonds, pumpkin seeds and peas, in your diet.

Symptoms of zinc deficiency include:

- white spots on nails
- low sperm count
- poor sense of taste
- poor sense of smell

You should take 30mg zinc a day.
Your partner should take 30mg zinc a day.

Selenium

Selenium is a mineral. As an antioxidant, it protects you against highly reactive chemical fragments called free radicals. These free radicals have been linked to cancer, coronary heart disease, rheumatoid arthritis and premature ageing. They speed up the ageing process by destroying healthy cells as well as attacking collagen (the 'cement' that holds cells together), which is found in bone, cartilage and connective tissues like skin.

Free radicals are created when oxygen becomes unstable during normal biochemical reactions in the body. They can also be formed by other sources, such as fried, blackened or barbecued food, radiation, exhaust fumes and smoking.

Antioxidants, such as selenium, are essential in your diet because they can disarm these harmful free radicals. With its protective effect, selenium can prevent chromosome breakage, which is known to be a cause of birth defects and miscarriages. It can also protect against poisoning from heavy toxic metals such as cadmium and lead (see pages 29 and 30) which can affect the development of sperm.

Good levels of selenium are essential to maximise sperm formation and are also needed for optimum testosterone production. In one double-blind trial, selenium supplementation resulted in an increase in fertility from 17.5 per cent to 35.1 per cent in subfertile men.[108]

Out of 41 men volunteering to be sperm donors in one study, 23 had normal sperm counts and 18 had low sperm counts. Blood selenium levels were significantly lower in the men with low sperm counts.[109]

Because selenium is needed for healthy sperm formation, it is especially advisable to supplement with selenium when semen analysis shows a high percentage of abnormal sperm. As a powerful antioxidant, selenium can also protect against possible DNA damage to sperm.

Selenium should be found in the soil where our food grows but unfortunately we can no longer rely on this. Because there are no obvious signs of deficiency, you don't know you're not getting enough until it is too late. It is therefore much safer to take a supplement.

You should take 100mcg of selenium a day.
Your partner should take 100mcg of selenium a day.

Essential Fatty Acids

The Department of Health recommends that we should all double our intake of Omega 3 oils by eating oily fish two to three times a week. This advice is based on the fact that, as their name implies, these oils are absolutely essential to good health.

Essential fats have a profound effect on every system of the body, including the reproductive system, and they are crucial for healthy hormone functioning. From these essential fatty acids you produce beneficial prostaglandins which have hormone-like functions. Endometriosis, which is a common problem that stops some women conceiving, involves an excess of some negative prostaglandins which can be controlled by adding in Omega 3 fatty acids from fish or linseed oil capsules. It is thought that fibroids (another condition that can affect fertility), also responds well to supplementing with these Omega 3 fatty acids.

For men essential fatty acid supplementation is crucial because the semen is rich in prostaglandins which are produced from these fats. When scientists have compared sperm samples from men with a good semen analysis, to those with problems such as abnormal sperm, poor motility or a low count, the semen in the poor samples lacks adequate levels of these beneficial prostaglandins.[110]

More and more research suggests that it is vital to supplement these fatty acids and not just rely on your dietary intake. Both you and your partner should start supplementing essential fatty acids three to four months before conception.

Because fish oil helps prevent blood from clotting inappropriately, supplementing with fish oil capsules can be beneficial to women who have recurrent miscarriages especially where the diagnosis has been linked to a clotting problem (see Section 5).[111]

So important are these essential fats that scientists have also looked at their role in pregnancy. They have found that they are crucial for brain, eyes and central nervous system development in the growing baby.[112]

They are also believed to prevent low birthweight and decrease the likelihood of a premature birth with all its inherent risks, including cerebral palsy, blindness, deafness, etc.[113]

As these essential fatty acids are so vital, it is advisable to supplement them in your diet in their most readily absorbable form. You can get GLA (Omega 6) from evening primrose, borage, blackcurrant or starflower. Whichever supplement you choose, read the GLA content on the back of the container and aim for a supplement that gives you at least 150mg of GLA per day. With EPA (Omega 3), aim for a supplement that will give you at least 300mg per day.

WARNING

Don't supplement with cod liver oil capsules. In the sea, fish can accumulate toxins and mercury, which pass through the liver, the organ of detoxification. Oil taken from the liver is therefore likely to give higher quantities of these toxins than oil taken from the body of the fish. Buy fish oil capsules from companies, like BioCare, that regularly check their fish oil supplements for contamination.

If you are vegetarian or prefer not to take fish oil, the other way to get Omega 3 fatty acids is by taking linseed oil capsules. Linseed oil contains both Omega 3 and Omega 6 essential fatty acids.

You should take 1000mg linseed oil
or 150mg GLA **and** 300mg EPA a day.

Your partner should take 1000mg linseed oil
or 150mg GLA **and** 300mg EPA a day.

B Vitamins

The B vitamins are water-soluble which means you lose them when passing urine.

Vitamin B6

Research has shown that giving B6 to women who have trouble conceiving increases their fertility. In one study a group of women who had stopped having periods because of a hormone imbalance were given vitamin B6 for three to four months. Some of the women started to have regular periods again.[114]

And in another study, 12 out of 14 women who had been trying for up to seven years conceived after taking vitamin B6 daily over six months.[115]

You should take up to 50mg a day.
Your partner should take up to 50mg a day.

Vitamin B12

Vitamin B12 is vital for cellular reproduction and a number of studies have shown its potential for increasing male fertility.[116] In one study in the 1980s, men with low sperm counts were given vitamin B12 each day and over a quarter of them improved by more than five times.[117]

You should take up to 50mcg a day.
Your partner should take up to 50mcg a day.

Vitamin E

Vitamin E is another powerful antioxidant. Like selenium, it plays a protective role in the body and benefits both male and female fertility.

With some couples, the woman is ovulating so her tubes are not blocked, and the man is producing a good quantity of sperm, yet the sperm cannot penetrate the egg, so there is no fertilisation. This is obviously a major problem and, in cases of poor fertilisation, even where the sperm count is good, doctors may have to resort to ICSI (see Chapter 19).

However, an intriguing piece of research looked at men who had good sperm counts but low fertilisation rates during IVF treatments. These men were given vitamin E each day. One month after starting treatment, the fertilisation rate had increased from 19 per cent to 29 per cent. These findings suggest that the antioxidant activity of vitamin E may make sperm more fertile.[118]

Like other antioxidants, vitamin E combats free radicals. (Linked to cancer, coronary heart disease, rheumatoid arthritis and premature ageing, free radicals speed up the ageing process by destroying healthy cells.) High levels of free radicals in semen can cause subfertility so it is important that any sperm problems are corrected by ensuring an adequate intake of antioxidants.[119]

If you have been told you have unexplained infertility I would recommend that you and your partner take vitamin E supplements. And if you have had a miscarriage you should take a vitamin E supplement because it prevents abnormal clotting.

One study, published in 1960, showed that giving vitamin E to both partners resulted in a significant increase in fertility.[120]

If you are over 35, and have been told that your fertility problems are caused by your age, then you are also likely to benefit from taking vitamin E. Studies show that adding antioxidants, such as vitamin C and vitamin E, to an animal's diet significantly reduces age-related ovulation decline. Another study concluded that 'these findings may have direct implications for preventing or delaying maternal-age-associated infertility in humans'.[121]

NATURAL OR SYNTHETIC VITAMIN E?

Natural and synthetic vitamins are normally of equal value because their molecular structures are identical. Vitamin E, however, is unusual because the natural and synthetic forms are structurally different.

Scientists have now tested to see what effect this difference has on the body. And it seems that natural vitamin E is more biologically active than the synthetic version, which means that the body utilises natural vitamin E more easily and it is retained for longer in body tissue, enabling it to perform its protective role.

A study in the *American Journal of Clinical Nutrition*, which looked at the effect of giving pregnant women both natural and synthetic vitamin E at the same time, found that the absorption rates of the two kinds of vitamin E were very different. The amount of natural vitamin E in the mother's blood was double that of the synthetic kind. And in the placental cords at delivery, there was three and a half times the amount of natural vitamin E as compared to the synthetic version. This means that natural vitamin E works more efficiently.

When you buy vitamin E, you want to get the most from the supplement, so you should choose the natural version, known as d-alpha-tocopherol, and avoid the synthetic one which is called dl-alpha-tocopherol.

You should take 300–400iu a day.
Your partner should take 300–400iu a day.

Vitamin C

Nearly all animals make vitamin C in their bodies, except humans, guinea pigs, fruit-eating bats, primates, the red-vented bulbul bird and the teleost fish! We have to get it all from our diet.

Studies have established that vitamin C enhances sperm quality. As a powerful antioxidant, it can protect the sperm and its DNA from damage.[122]

In one study a group of men had their vitamin C intake deliberately reduced from 250mg a day to 5mg a day. Their sperm had double the normal DNA damage.[123] (We do not yet know for sure but it is possible that certain types of DNA damage make it difficult to conceive in the first place or cause an increased risk of miscarriage or a chromosome problem in the developing baby.)

When sperm stick together (agglutinate), this can obviously reduce the chances of conceiving. Yet research has shown that sometimes as little as 500mg of vitamin C per day can help prevent this.[124]

Some placebo-controlled trials (where some of the men were given a 'dummy' pill instead of vitamin C) have shown that supplementing with 1000mg of vitamin C per day increased sperm counts, improved motility and reduced the percentage of abnormal sperm.[125]

If a woman isn't ovulating she is usually given the drug clomiphene to stimulate ovulation (see Section 4). Sometimes the drug does not work and there is still no ovulation. But it appears that if vitamin C is taken at the same time as the clomiphene it can help trigger ovulation.[126]

You may have been worried by newspaper scare stories claiming that vitamin C could 'promote cancer'. These were actually due to the press misinterpreting the findings of a preliminary investigation.[127] In fact, the study to assess the effect of vitamin C on cellular damage drew very conflicting conclusions and attracted criticism from the scientific world which felt that 'the conclusions were not justified by the data'.[128]

In any event, one piece of research should always be weighed against other existing research. In this case numerous other studies have demonstrated the beneficial effects of supplementing with good levels of vitamin C.

You should take 1000mg a day.
Your partner should take 1000mg a day.

Manganese

Manganese, an essential trace element, is needed for healthy skin, bone and cartilage formation and to regulate blood sugar levels. It also plays a part in cell protection because it helps to activate an enzyme called superoxide dismutase (SOD). SOD is an important antioxidant enzyme because it protects the mitochondria (microscopic structures containing genetic material found in cells) from free radical attack.

Research has shown that women with low manganese levels are more likely to give birth to a baby with a malformation.[129]

You should take 5mg a day.
Your partner should take 5mg a day.

Iron

We need iron to make red blood cells and to transport oxygen around our bodies. Without iron, new cells could not be produced and our organs would be starved of oxygen. The negative side is that we do not eliminate iron; it is continually stored as ferritin. The only time we lose iron is during a period, childbirth, an accident causing blood-loss, or by donating blood. Iron is part of haemoglobin, the oxygen-carrying component of the blood. A deficiency of iron causes tiredness, because the body is being starved of oxygen.

Iron deficiency should always be checked during infertility investigations, as taking iron is known to have helped women regain their fertility.[130]

Iron supplements, given together with vitamin C (which increases the absorption of iron), have resulted in a number of women with fertility problems becoming pregnant, including one woman who had undergone nine years of unsuccessful fertility treatment.[131]

Scientists used to believe that the more iron we had, the better. Years ago iron supplements were given routinely during pregnancy, regardless of whether the woman had a deficiency or not. Thankfully, this practice has now stopped.

You should only take iron if you know you have a deficiency and your doctor can test you for this. Heavy periods (menorrhagia) can cause iron deficiency because of the excessive blood loss but, ironically, iron deficiency can also cause heavy periods.[132]

The most absorbable form of iron, haem iron, is found in animal products such as fish and poultry. Non-haem iron is found in leafy green vegetables and dried fruit. Vegetarians can have smaller iron stores because the iron in the food they eat is less absorbable.[133]

Apart from eating iron-rich foods, you can increase your iron intake by *not* drinking tea with food. This is because the tannin contained in tea can block the uptake of iron, as well as other vital minerals. You need to leave at least an hour between eating and then drinking tea, or, better still, eliminate it altogether because of the known effects of caffeine on fertility.

Your choice of cooking utensils can also affect your iron intake. For example, cooking acidic foods, such as tomatoes, in an iron pan can be a source of dietary iron; and studies show that cooking any food in an iron pot can increase iron intake.[134]

Aluminium, on the other hand, can actually diminish the iron content of food. Conversely, cooking in stainless steel has also been shown to significantly increase the iron content of food.[135]

Symptoms of iron deficiency include:

- Fatigue
- Sore tongue
- Cracks at the side of the mouth
- Vertical ridges on the finger nails
- Spoon-shaped (concave) nails
- Hair loss or poor hair growth
- Breathlessness
- Pale complexion

NOT ALL IRON SUPPLEMENTS ARE THE SAME

If you are found to be deficient in iron, you will probably be given a supplement to take. Unfortunately, some iron supplements are ineffective, depending on the form in which they are given.

Inorganic iron, such as ferrous sulphate and ferrous gluconate (the standard irons given medically), is very difficult to absorb and can cause digestive problems, resulting in constipation or black stools. Inorganic iron or chelated forms of iron (which are combined with an amino acid) are much more easily absorbed and do not usually cause any bowel changes. Ask for the latter.

Iron supplements should only be taken if a blood test shows a deficiency.

L-Arginine

L-arginine is an amino acid found in many foods. The head of the sperm contains an exceptional amount of this nutrient which is essential for sperm production. As long ago as 1944, researchers found that an arginine-free diet – even for just a few days – prevented sperm maturing correctly.[136]

Since then, a great deal of research has shown that L-arginine supplementation should be considered seriously when there are problems with sperm and male fertility.[137] According to one study, supplementing with L-arginine can help to increase both the sperm count and quality.[138] Other research showed that sperm counts doubled after supplementation and there was also an increase in the number of pregnancies.[139]

> **WARNING**
>
> People who have herpes attacks (either cold sores or genital herpes) should not supplement arginine because it stimulates the virus.

Your partner should take 1000mg a day.

L-Carnitine

Another amino acid called L-carnitine also appears to be essential for normal functioning of sperm cells. High levels of L-carnitine have been found in sperm cells and it seems the higher the level, the better the sperm count and motility.[140]

Supplementing with L-carnitine over four months helped to increase the number of normal sperm in men with a high percentage of abnormal forms,[141] and to increase their sperm count.[142]

Your partner should take 100mg a day.

Vitamin A

This vitamin deserves special mention because there is a lot of confusion about its use before and during pregnancy. The key point is that it is important to have good amounts of vitamin A at the point of conception because it is essential to the developing embryo.

Recently, concerns have been raised about the use of vitamin A while trying to become pregnant and during pregnancy. These problems were brought to light by a number of women who regularly ate large amounts of liver during pregnancy. (In the past, women were told to eat liver when pregnant because it is a good source of iron. However, liver also contains large amounts of the animal form of vitamin A, retinol, and it is this that appears to cause the problems.)

A study in the *New England Journal of Medicine* found that pregnant women who take high doses of retinol every day increase their risk of having a handicapped baby. The danger threshold appears to be daily doses in excess of 10,000iu, which results in a one in 57 chance of having a handicapped baby (compared to those who take just half that dose).

Interestingly, it seems that vegetable sources of vitamin A (beta-carotene) do not cause any defects in an unborn child so eating carrots, tomatoes, cabbage, spinach and broccoli is much safer than eating animal sources of vitamin A.[143]

One of the dangers of giving health advice is that the public reacts by swinging from one extreme to another. This has been the case with vitamin A because the usual recommendation now is to take no vitamin A during pregnancy. Yet the consequences of a deficiency of vitamin A during pregnancy can be just as devastating.

Vitamin A has antioxidant and protective properties similar to those of selenium, which protect against cell mutation. It is essential for healthy eyes and, in animal studies, a deficiency of vitamin A has produced newborn animals with no eyes, eye defects, undescended testes and diaphragmatic hernias.[144]

BENEFITS OF VITAMIN A IN PREGNANCY

In developing nations, deaths in pregnant women are far from rare and may be as much as 50 to 100 times higher than in industrialised countries. And yet studies show that by taking 42mg of beta-carotene daily, this death rate can be reduced by 49 per cent. By taking vitamin A, as retinol, there can be a reduction of 40 per cent.[145]

You should take up to 2500iu of Vitamin A a day.

Choosing Your Supplements

I can hear you wondering how you and your partner are going to manage to take all these supplements. Well, it's not as difficult as you might think. You should first find a multivitamin and mineral supplement designed for pregnancy. There are plenty on the market – good makes that I would recommend are BioCare, Solgar and Foresight and also Fertility Plus (see Section 6 for details of structuring a supplement programme).

A special pregnancy supplement like these will include the 400mcg of folic acid you need each day as well as a safe level of vitamin A so you should not need to add these in separately.

Then see what else is in the supplement. You should find that most of the other recommendations are included and the label will give you the amounts. If the amounts are less than those I have recommended (see below) then you should take a separate supplement to 'top up' those nutrients.

So, for example, if the multivitamin and mineral contains 50mcg of selenium you will need to supplement with an extra 50mcg to reach your total of 100mcg.

Your partner should also find a good multivitamin and mineral supplement, such as Fertility Plus for Men – and then top up with the extras in the same way.

Summary of required doses in supplements

Nutrient	You	Your partner
folic acid	400mcg	–
zinc	30mg	30mg
selenium	100mcg	100mcg
linseed oil *or*	1000mg	1000mg
GLA *and*	150mg	150mg
EPA	300mg	300mg
vitamin B6	up to 50mg	up to 50mg
vitamin B12	up to 50mcg	up to 50mcg
vitamin E	300–400iu	300–400iu
vitamin C	1000mg	1000mg
vitamin A	up to 2500iu	–
manganese	5mg	5mg
iron	if needed	–
L-arginine		1000mg
L-carnitine		100mg

Conclusion

As you can see these nutrients offer us a great many benefits. And the benefits of many more nutrients in relation to fertility have yet to be discovered.

This is why it is so important to have a varied diet – in order to ensure that you get many different nutrients. The table below shows which foods are particularly rich in these essential vitamins and minerals. But in these days of refined foods, I believe it is important to take supplements to make up any shortfalls in your diet. None the less, as their name implies, food supplements are supplementary to your diet; they are not a substitute for good food. So, don't assume that you can eat junk foods and take supplements and still be in the best of health.

There is a tendency for certain vitamins and minerals to be hyped in the press. So often, a certain nutrient or vitamin suddenly becomes the fashionable answer to virtually every problem on the planet. This is nonsense. In nature all nutrients work together and many are dependent on each other to function properly. So it is important when thinking about supplements – whatever your situation – to take a good multivitamin and mineral supplement as the basic foundation and then add in other individual nutrients on top.

Case History

Sarah was 34 when she came to see me for preconception care. She had been born with spina bifida and had been told that she had a one in seven chance of having a baby with it too. In this situation I needed to make sure she was taking 5mg of folic acid before conception rather than the standard 400mcg.

I sent her for an infection test which showed that she had a number of infections including Group B haemolytic streptococcus. She was treated for these and then given an intensive course of acidophilus to recolonise her gut. Her mineral levels showed deficiencies in selenium and zinc with high levels of lead. Her partner had extremely low levels of zinc and was also deficient in calcium and selenium. He was showing high levels of both aluminium and lead. They followed the Four-Month Plan (see Section 6) in order to correct these deficiencies and I gave them both extra antioxidants to bring down the lead and aluminium over the four months. They now have a healthy baby girl.

Convincing Your Partner

Your partner may wonder if it is worth going to all this trouble of changing lifestyle habits, eliminating alcohol and taking supplements. But there is a real bonus for him because his general health will almost certainly improve. Many men report that they have more energy, fewer headaches, better digestion and feel more relaxed, and that other health problems that may have dogged them have cleared up. For instance, one man who consulted me with his wife when they had problems conceiving found that the changes I recommended to improve his fertility also cleared up a very upsetting skin complaint he suffered from called psoriasis. He said he had been to the best dermatologists and psoriasis experts and no-one had managed to achieve these results. It cleared up because the actual foundation of his health was improved by these simple and yet effective lifestyle and dietary changes.

And there is real evidence that this programme can transform your partner's fertility. This is what happened when one man followed the recommendations to boost his fertility. The semen samples were taken three months apart and show a very significant improvement in a short space of time:

	28/03/99	25/06/99
Total sperm count	15 million/ml	125 million/ml
Sperm active and progressing well	5%	45%
Normal sperm	5%	40%

This is an example of how striking the difference can be, even after only a short time.

Dietary sources of nutrients

Nutrient	Good food sources
zinc	oysters (maybe some of those so-called myths about oysters being an aphrodisiac do have some scientific basis), pumpkin seeds, wholewheat, rye, oats, almonds, peas
selenium	tuna, sesame seeds, shellfish, avocados and wholegrains
vitamin E	oily fish (like tuna, sardines and salmon), sesame seeds, peanuts, and unrefined oils (including corn and sunflower oil)
vitamin C	raw peppers, broccoli, cauliflower, strawberries, peas, baked potatoes, oranges
L-arginine	dairy, poultry, fish and nuts
vitamin A	carrots, tomatoes, cabbage, spinach and broccoli

Case History

Deirdre and her partner were both 31 when they came to see me because Deirdre's irregular cycles, some as long as 41 days, were making it hard to conceive. Her Body Mass Index (see page 58) was also only 17 so I explained the link between being underweight and fertility and asked her to put on weight. She was also low in zinc and selenium. Deirdre's partner had only a third of the required level of zinc and also low levels of selenium and magnesium. His first semen analysis showed a count of 25 million but 84 per cent of the sperm were abnormal, 75 per cent were not moving at all, and only 5 per cent were moving normally.

But within three months of going on the Preconception Plan (see Section 6), his sperm count had risen to 106 million and the quality of the sperm had improved dramatically, with 50 per cent of them moving normally. The couple then went on a maintenance programme of supplements and kept up the changes in diet and lifestyle and they conceived a month later and now have a healthy baby boy.

CHAPTER 11

Exploring Complementary Medical Approaches

Alongside the lifestyle and dietary changes described in this section of the book, you may find it helpful to try one or more complementary approaches, such as herbal medicine, homeopathy or acupuncture.

Herbal Medicine

Herbs are the oldest form of medicine and have been used for healing all over the world. Reproduction and the rites surrounding it have always had a central role in traditional cultures so it is not surprising that herbal medicine is particularly rich in effective remedies for fertility problems.

Herbs are in fact the foundation of numerous pharmaceutical drugs. For instance, aspirin is based on an extract from willow, originally used for pain relief by Native Americans. Up to 70 per cent of drugs in use today have their origins in plants. But modern drug companies only use the active ingredient of the plant or herb, while ancient peoples always used (and still use) the whole plant. The advantage of using the whole plant is that the side-effects are absent or minimal. That is the big difference between modern and herbal medicine.

In traditional times, for instance, the foxglove plant (*digitalis purpurea*) was used for heart problems. In modern times, scientists have isolated the main active ingredient of the foxglove (digoxin) and put it into tablet form but in so doing have created a real risk of side-effects. By using the whole plant, the active ingredient interacts with all the other constituents of the plant which naturally include 'buffer' ingredients that counteract any side-effect. Herbalists believe this is the proper way to use the healing powers of herbs and plants.

The easiest and most effective way of taking herbs is in tincture form, using approximately 5ml (1 teaspoon) three times daily in a little water. Try to get tinctures made from organically grown herbs. In the liquid form the herbs are already dissolved. They are therefore absorbed faster so their action is quicker. In the dry form, the tablets or capsules have to be digested and the benefit of the herbs is only as good as your own digestive and absorption processes. Herbs are not like drugs. If drugs are stopped, the symptoms can return and you are back where you started. The herbs stop the symptoms but they are also addressing the cause at the same time, so the symptoms are being alleviated because the body is becoming more balanced.

The particular herbs listed below have proved very effective in balancing hormones and boosting both male and female fertility and conception rates.

Agnus Castus (Vitex/chasteberry)

This is a popular herb which grows in Mediterranean countries and central Asia. It does not contain any hormones but it stimulates the function of the pituitary gland which controls and balances our hormones by producing luteinising hormone. This increases progesterone production and helps regulate a woman's cycle. Agnus castus also helps keep prolactin secretion in check.[146] (Excessive prolactin can prevent ovulation.)

This herb has been used by women who had established luteal phase defect (shortened second half of the cycle) and high prolactin levels. In one study 48 women diagnosed with infertility took agnus castus daily for three months.[147] Seven of them became pregnant during that time and 25 of them regained normal progesterone levels.

Agnus castus works to restore hormonal balance and can be used where there are hormone deficits as well as excesses. It:

- regulates periods
- restarts periods which have stopped
- helps with heavy bleeding
- helps with too-frequent periods
- helps with painful periods
- increases the ratio of progesterone to oestrogen by balancing excess oestrogen

I have seen a number of women who needed to have IVF treatment but could not do so because their levels of Follicle Stimulating Hormone (FSH) were too high. The highest FSH level for most IVF treatments is 10, and rising FSH levels can indicate a pre-menopausal condition. The use of agnus castus, sometimes with a mix of other herbs, brought down the FSH level so that the women could go for IVF treatment.

Dong Quai (Angelica Sinensis)

This is an Oriental herb frequently used for menstrual complaints. It is extensively cultivated in Asia for medicinal purposes and in traditional Chinese medicine is well-known as a tonic for the female reproductive system. It:

- tones a weak uterus
- regulates irregular periods
- alleviates period pains
- reduces spotting
- helps with absent periods

False Unicorn Root (Chamaelirium Luteum)

This North American herb is a good tonic and strengthener for the reproductive system and can be used for both men and women, as it has a balancing effect on hormones. Herbalists often give it to women after a miscarriage or an infection in the pelvic area. Mixed with other herbs, it can be given for ovarian cysts or endometriosis. It is also used to try and prevent a threatened miscarriage. It:

- balances the hormones
- regularises delayed periods
- regularises absent periods

Saw Palmetto (Serenoa Serrulate)

This is one of the best herbs for the male reproductive system. It acts like a tonic for the man and has traditionally been used for centuries to treat enlarged prostate.

Using Herbs

If you have a specific ailment, like polycystic ovaries or endometriosis, you should consult a good herbalist or health professional with experience in using herbs so that the remedy can be tailored to your individual needs. (To find a practitioner, see Useful Addresses on page 229.)

If you have been told that you have a hormone imbalance or your cycles are irregular then it is worth taking the herb agnus castus over a few months, as this is a good balancing herb. It is an adaptogen which means that, whether you suffer from a low level of one hormone or an excess of a different one, you can take agnus castus and achieve normal levels. Buy an organic tincture of agnus castus and take 1 teaspoon three times a day for three or four months or until you conceive.

WARNING

Herbs have to be used with caution once you are pregnant. There are some that are especially useful in the late stages of pregnancy (raspberry leaf, for example). But, once you are pregnant, it is important only to take herbs with professional advice. If you are actually having medical hormonal treatment for fertility you should stop taking herbs but keep taking the nutritional supplements.

Case History

Susan and her partner were 30 and 31 and had been trying to have a baby for four years before they came to see me. They had been told they had unexplained fertility and had four unsuccessful attempts at IUI (see page 163). Susan had a lot of problems with her periods. She had a regular cycle but had heavy bleeding with spotting and headaches before her period and at ovulation her abdomen would swell up and she would feel sick.

I asked them to be screened for any infections and the test came back positive to one infection so they both took antibiotics and were then re-tested to make sure they were all clear. Susan was deficient in a number of nutrients, including zinc, selenium, calcium and magnesium, and her partner had low zinc and high aluminium levels. I therefore recommended that he cut out canned drinks and switch to an aluminium-free deodorant. I also used a combination of balancing herbs such as agnus castus to alleviate Susan's spotting and heavy bleedings, as I was concerned that the imbalance causing the problem with Susan's cycle was also a factor in her inability to conceive. Susan and her partner followed the Four-Month Plan outlined in Section 6 and waited until their mineral levels were back to normal. Nine months from their first appointment they conceived.

Homeopathy

The word homeopathy comes from the Greek words *homos* (meaning 'same') and *pathos* (meaning 'suffering'). In homeopathy different people suffering from the same problem can be given different remedies because each person is treated according to their individual constitution. Pulsatilla is often given for women with no periods or irregular periods.[148] General remedies recommended for male infertility could include lycopodium, argentum nitricum and selenium metallicum. Because infertility is multifactorial, it is better to consult a qualified homeopath so that the treatment is individualised. Specific help could be given for endometriosis, fibroids, cysts and other complaints. (See Useful Addresses on page 229 for advice on how to contact a homeopathic practitioner.)

Acupuncture

Acupuncture can also be used alongside the other recommendations in this book to help increase fertility. It is an ancient system of Chinese medicine that dates back some 2,000 years and is based on the concept of Qi (pronounced 'chee') which is the body's energy. The acupuncturist aims to balance this flow of Qi along pathways called meridians. Acupuncture has proved particularly successful in boosting the fertility of older women who want to get pregnant. Chinese herbs may also be given with acupuncture and an interesting study on infertile women at Qian Fo Shan Hospital in Jinan, China, showed a pregnancy rate within two years of 70 per cent for those given acupuncture, 52.7 per cent with herbs and 46.7 per cent with conventional drugs. Acupuncture can be especially useful for correcting hormonal imbalances and problems such as fibroids and endometriosis.

Conclusion

Don't feel that you must have all the above treatments. The most important factor is nutrition and this should be your prime focus because you *are* what you eat. If you follow the recommendations in the previous chapter, this should be enough to make a major difference. If you would like extra help then choose the therapy that most appeals to you and that you can afford – they are not available on the NHS. I have had most success combining nutrition and herbs.

CHAPTER 12

Having Yourself Tested for Nutritional Deficiencies and Toxins

Now you have seen how a shortage of different nutrients can reduce your fertility as a couple. And, more importantly, you have seen how a few simple changes can dramatically improve your chances of having a healthy baby. But how would you actually know if you had a nutrient deficiency?

Most of us are short of time these days. We snatch a sandwich for lunch, often on the move, and maybe have not been eating so well over the last few years. With our food being depleted in nutrients because of the way it has been processed and the impoverishment of the soil it is grown on, the chances are that many of us are deficient in some nutrients.

It is very easy to pick up a newspaper or magazine and read how wonderful zinc or selenium is, and then go out and buy some. But this is a very random approach. It is much better to be tested so that you know you are taking the nutrients you really need. The vitamins and minerals you need for your body to function at its optimum and give you the best chance of conceiving are all dependent on each other in order to act efficiently. For instance, zinc works best when it is accompanied by adequate amounts of vitamin B6 so it is better to take a combined multivitamin and mineral supplement and then add the extra nutrients that you are deficient in.

The other reason for testing is that all the chemicals and other toxic substances we absorb in our daily life can collect in our systems and damage our fertility. We need to check this out too.

Hair Analysis

There are many ways of testing nutritional status – using samples of blood or sweat, for instance. But one of the most cost-effective and convenient ways is through a hair sample. Hair has been shown to reflect a good long-term record of our mineral and nutritional experience.[149]

Eventually hair samples could be used to screen for potential diabetes or breast cancer. Work is being undertaken in Australia by Professor Veronica James at the University of New South Wales where hair is being analysed with a technique called X-ray diffraction. As X-rays are fired through the hair they form a pattern on photographic film. From this pattern the researchers are able to pick up different information. For instance, with hair from a diabetic patient, sugar binds onto the hair filaments. It will therefore look different from a strand of hair taken from a person without diabetes.

Hair samples can also be used to test for drug use, such as cocaine, amphetamines and cannabis. This is helpful in forensic medicine and pathology, for example to determine whether somebody was under the influence of drugs in an accident.

Because your hair cells are some of the fastest-growing cells in your body, they can 'lock in' information about your exposure to certain nutrients as they grow. In this way, your hair forms a permanent record of your exposure to beneficial and toxic elements. Analysing hair is therefore also an excellent way to test for heavy toxic metals and is used in many medical studies to assess exposure to metals like mercury.[150]

Other ways of testing, with blood or urine for instance, can be less reliable, because the results are influenced by what you may have eaten. Also your body tries to keep everything in balance. To do this, it tops up the levels of nutrients in your blood by taking them from elsewhere. For instance, if your blood calcium levels fall your body will pinch calcium from your bones to keep the level constant. A blood test may then suggest that your calcium levels are fine. But a hair analysis showing high levels of calcium would help identify the leeching of calcium from your bones.

However, like any testing method, hair analysis has its limitations. For instance, when testing for nutrients it is important that your hair is not contaminated by tints, highlights or perms. Certain minerals (iron, for instance) are best tested by blood samples. But levels of trace elements can be higher in hair, which make them easier to analyse. Also, because hair doesn't need specialised sampling equipment or storage, this form of testing is accessible for couples who don't live near a qualified practitioner.

Hair can be used to analyse your levels of calcium, magnesium, zinc, selenium, copper, manganese, chromium and also the toxic metals mercury, aluminium and cadmium.

The minerals are usually analysed, together with a detailed questionnaire.

Then a personalised programme of supplements is recommended for you and your partner. This programme should be followed for a minimum of four months and then the hair should be re-tested.

Once your mineral and toxic levels are back to normal, you will be given a maintenance programme to follow until you become pregnant (see Section 6).

In the twelfth week of pregnancy, you will be tested again. Your nutrient needs during pregnancy are different and your programme will be adjusted accordingly. You should then continue with the amended programme until you have your baby.

If your starting levels of nutrients were very deficient or your toxic metal levels extremely high then you should stay on the programme for longer.

If you are planning to have fertility treatment (see Section 4), you should follow the programme for four months beforehand. This will ensure that the egg and sperm are as healthy as they can be before treatment starts, to give the procedure the best possible chance of working.

Mineral analysis can also identify substances that reduce your and your partner's fertility. For example, if you have used the pill or an IUD (coil) you may have high levels of copper. This can also be due to fertility treatment, where the drugs used increase copper levels. High levels of copper are a concern, as they are often matched by low zinc levels which can dramatically affect levels of fertility and may also give an increased rate of miscarriage.[151]

WARNING

If you are a keen swimmer this can confuse the analysis because the pools are treated with algicides which increase the copper levels in your hair.

You and your partner may turn out to have high levels of copper and other toxic metals and this may well explain your fertility problems.

The results of the mineral tests are given to you in the form of a graph so that you can see how far your levels differ from the norm (see opposite).

Results of hair mineral analysis test before treatment

(ALL RESULTS IN PARTS PER MILLION)

	REFERENCE RANGE	RESULTS		LOW		REFERENCE RANGE		HIGH	
CALCIUM	200 – 600	538							Ca
MAGNESIUM	30 – 95	27							Mg
PHOSPHORUS*	100 – 210	117							P
SODIUM*	90 – 340	514							Na
POTASSIUM*	50 – 120	67							K
IRON*	20 – 60	30							Fe
COPPER	10 – 40	27							Cu
ZINC	150 – 240	137							Zn
CHROMIUM	0.60 – 1.50	0.76							Cr
MANGANESE	1.0 – 2.6	1.1							Mn
SELENIUM	1.5 – 4.0	1.5							Se
NICKEL	0.40 – 1.40	0.67							Ni
COBALT*	0.10 – 0.70	0.24							Co

* Clinical significance of hair concentration of asterisked elements has not been established.

	ACCEPT	RAISED	TOXIC	RESULT		ACCEPTABLE		RAISED		TOXIC	
LEAD	<15.0	15.0 – 40.0	>40.0	4.1							Pb
MERCURY	<2.0	2.0 – 5.0	>5.0	0.37							Hg
CADMIUM	<0.5	0.5 – 2.0	>2.0	0.53							Cd
ARSENIC	<2.0	2.0 – 5.0	>5.0	0.24							As
ALUMINIUM	<10.0	10.0 – 25.0	>25.0	2.1							Al

Results of hair mineral analysis test after treatment

(ALL RESULTS IN PARTS PER MILLION)

	REFERENCE RANGE	RESULTS		LOW		REFERENCE RANGE		HIGH	
CALCIUM	200 – 600	516							Ca
MAGNESIUM	30 – 95	46							Mg
PHOSPHORUS*	100 – 210	170							P
SODIUM*	90 – 340	220							Na
POTASSIUM*	50 – 120	78							K
IRON*	20 – 60	21							Fe
COPPER	10 – 40	27							Cu
ZINC	150 – 240	193							Zn
CHROMIUM	0.60 – 1.50	0.71							Cr
MANGANESE	1.0 – 2.6	1.4							Mn
SELENIUM	1.5 – 4.0	2.2							Se
NICKEL	0.40 – 1.40	0.71							Ni
COBALT*	0.10 – 0.70	0.19							Co

* Clinical significance of hair concentration of asterisked elements has not been established.

	ACCEPT	RAISED	TOXIC	RESULT		ACCEPTABLE		RAISED		TOXIC	
LEAD	<15.0	15.0 – 40.0	>40.0	3.9							Pb
MERCURY	<2.0	2.0 – 5.0	>5.0	0.40							Hg
CADMIUM	<0.5	0.5 – 2.0	>2.0	0.17							Cd
ARSENIC	<2.0	2.0 – 5.0	>5.0	0.16							As
ALUMINIUM	<10.0	10.0 – 25.0	>25.0	1.6							Al

The two hair mineral analysis charts above show the difference before and after taking food supplements. In the first chart the patient has lower levels of magnesium, zinc and selenium, and her cadmium level is too high as a result of smoking. In the second chart, after taking an appropriate supplement programme, her mineral levels are back to normal and the cadmium is reduced (she gave up smoking too).

What To Do

First you must try and work out the source of contamination and avoid it if possible. Then you must take specific nutrients, such as antioxidants, which will help eliminate the toxins from your body.

Avoiding Toxic Metals

Look at Chapter 5 to check if your or your partner's work exposes you to the toxic metals shown up by hair analysis. If your occupation has been ruled out as the cause then look at other possibilities:

- **Lead** – traffic fumes from living by a main road or cycling to work, lead waterpipes?

- **Mercury** – recent dental work or a lot of previous dental work, high intake of canned tuna fish?

- **Cadmium** – from smoking and also from exposure to passive smoke?

- **Aluminium** – indigestion tablets, aluminium cookware or foil, canned drinks, dried milk substitutes, deodorants?

Vitamin C is very useful in helping to eliminate toxins from the body, and you and your partner should be taking it each day as part of your supplement programme. But you can do much more to rid your system of unwanted substances by toning up your liver. This is a vital gland (the largest in the body) which acts as a marvellous disposal unit for toxins and waste products when it is working efficiently.

The liver detoxifies by combining harmful substances (like chemicals, drugs, alcohol and heavy toxic metals) with less harmful substances which are then excreted by the kidneys. So making sure your liver is working efficiently will not only help eliminate heavy metals but will also help rid your body of pesticide residues and other unwanted substances.

Taking Detoxifying Herbs

Herbs can be extremely helpful in optimising liver function and one of the best is milk thistle (*Silybum marianum*). This herb can increase the number of new liver cells that are produced to replace old damaged ones.[152] Silymarin is the collective name for the substances found in milk thistle which have this beneficial effect.

Conclusion

You may want to have a personal consultation with a nutritional practitioner so that tests can be organised and your plan of action can be structured to your own individual needs. If you do not have a nutritional therapist near you (see British Association of Nutritional Therapists under Useful Addresses), then you are welcome to get in touch with me (see Staying in Touch, page 242) and a postal consultation can be arranged.

CHAPTER 13

*Protecting Yourself Against
Environmental and
Occupational Hazards*

We now know that certain pollutants and chemicals in the environment can affect both male and female fertility, and there may be many more substances that we come into contact with in everyday life that combine to form a 'toxic cocktail' with unknown long-term consequences.

The problem is that these suspect substances seem to be absolutely everywhere – in the food we eat, the air we breathe, and the things we use at work and at home. We can avoid many of them, and minimise our exposure to others. But we obviously cannot completely eliminate them, short of finding a non-polluted desert island to go and live on.

However, reducing your exposure is only part of the plan. There are plenty of ways to fortify yourself and your partner against the effects of unavoidable exposure and to ensure that toxins are successfully eliminated from your system. In my experience, dramatic results have been achieved by couples whose 'unexplained fertility' turns out to have been due to exposure to some of these substances.

Xenoestrogens

These are synthetic oestrogens which affect the fertility of wildlife and are causing some animals to grow both male and female sex organs. They come from pesticides and plastics and are stored in body fat and can affect men and women differently.

The massive proliferation of xenoestrogens has coincided with:

- A decrease in sperm counts of 50 per cent over the last ten years.

- An increase in testicular cancer.

- Earlier onset of puberty. (At the turn of the century the average age was 15. Now some girls as young as eight are growing breasts and pubic hair. It has been found that girls can enter puberty almost a year earlier if their pregnant mothers had higher levels of two synthetic chemicals, PCBs and DDE, while they were pregnant.)[153]

- A doubling in the number of boys born with undescended testes (which means they may not produce sperm) between 1962 and 1981.[154]

- Increasing numbers of male babies born with problems with their penis. Some boys are born with the opening of the urethra (where urine passes out of the body) on the side of the penis instead of the top. In extreme cases male babies have been born with both male and female organs.[155]

Synthetic oestrogens, similar to those in use in the pesticides and plastics industry, have been linked to cancers and abnormalities.

Years ago women who suffered recurrent miscarriages were treated with a synthetic oestrogen called dithethylstilbestrol (DES). Now their grown-up daughters, who were exposed to DES in the womb, are showing high rates of cervical abnormalities that can lead to recurrent miscarriages or infertility. Some have developed a rare and sometimes fatal vaginal cancer (clear-cell adenocarcinoma). Their sons are not so severely affected but some have suffered mild genital abnormalities.

Further evidence comes from Professor Ana Soto in Boston, USA, who was studying breast cancer cells stored in large incubators. These cancer cells started to divide and multiply as if oestrogen was present. But when the laboratory changed the tubes on the incubators the cells stopped dividing. It turned out that nonylphenol, a synthetic oestrogen similar to those widely used in paints, toiletries, agricultural chemicals and detergents, had been used in the manufacture of the tubes.

In another example of the power of these chemicals, some male workers developed breasts after inhaling dust containing bisphenol A, a synthetic oestrogen used in a wide range of packaging (e.g. for soft drinks, bottled water and even babies' bottles).

Phthalates, found in PVC, food packaging and glues, are another class of chemical which has an oestrogen-like effect on humans.

Types of chemicals that affect hormone balance and fertility include:

- **Pesticides** (DDT, DDE, endosulfan, methoxychlor, heptachlor, toxaphene, dieldrin, lindane)

- **Plastic compounds** (Alkyphenols such as nonylphenol and octylphenol, biphenolic compounds such as bisphenol A, phthalates)

- **Pharmaceutical drugs** (Synthetic drugs like DES)

- **Industrial substances** (PCBs, dioxin)

In Your Food

The food we buy in the supermarket is produced by intensive methods of farming heavily dependent on the use of chemicals, and our government has little control over the levels of toxins it contains.

For instance, DDT is banned in the UK but it can enter our food chain through imported food. It is still detected in breast milk and is very hard to eliminate from the body.

In 1994, the British government found 'unexpectedly high residues of actually toxic pesticides in some individual carrots'. And in some cases, the amount of pesticide was three times the government's Acceptable Daily Intake (ADI).

There are 3,900 brands of insecticide, herbicide and fungicide approved for use in the UK. Some fruit and vegetables are sprayed *ten* times with chemicals before they reach the supermarket shelves. And huge amounts of chemicals can be used *after* harvesting. For example, green tomatoes are exposed to ethylene gas to turn them red. And fruit is dosed with chemicals such as carbendazium and metalaxl to stop it rotting before it gets to the shop. It can also be waxed to 'seal in' the chemicals.

Pesticides are also used during livestock production. And meat production is heavily dependent on antibiotics to stop intensively reared animals getting diseased. This overuse of antibiotics could cause an increase in devastating human diseases like TB and meningitis which are now becoming resistant to antibiotic treatment.

Food poisoning bugs (like salmonella and campylobacter), found in farm animals, are already becoming resistant to drug treatment. Penicillin use on UK farms has increased *eight* times in the last 30 years. In fact the amount of antibiotics used is higher than in human medicine.

The European Union has banned 19 antibiotics in animal feed because they are worried that the development of new drug-resistant super-bugs could kill humans. (Antibiotics pass through the animal's digestive system, through the milk, which is sold on for us to drink or to be made into cheese, yogurt or butter.)

US beef has been banned by the European Union because growth hormones given to cows in the US to increase milk yields are thought to be linked to breast and prostate cancers.

Additives and preservatives in prepared and processed food are listed as E numbers on labels. But European wine-labelling regulations forbid the listing of ingredients on the bottle. Fish bladders, sulphur, egg white and gelatine (made from animal bones) are just some of the substances that are apparently added to wine. And grapes may have received up to 14 applications of herbicides, pesticides and fungicides before they are made into wine.

What You Can Do

- Buy organic produce whenever possible. (When tested, organic farmers who farmed and ate vegetables without pesticides and chemical fertilisers had almost double the sperm count of men from other professions such as engineers and electricians.[156])
- Avoid, as far as possible, food and drinks in plastic containers or wrapped in plastic, especially fatty foods in plastic. This is because xenoestrogens are lipophilic (fat-loving) and will therefore migrate into foods like cheese and crisps. Remove food from plastic packaging as soon as possible. And reduce your own intake of saturated fats.
- Do not heat food in plastic especially in a microwave oven. (Scientists have discovered that clingfilm used in the microwave leaches damaging chemicals into the food.)
- If your vegetables and fruit are not organic, wash them thoroughly. You can buy a wash (like Veggi Wash) from your healthfood shop which claims to be able to remove farm chemicals, waxes and surface grime. Washing cannot alter the amount of pesticides inherently absorbed into the vegetables. But peeling fruit can lower the pesticide residues by about three-quarters.
- Increase your intake of fibre – it helps prevent the absorption of oestrogenic chemicals into the bloodstream. Fibre is found in wholegrains, vegetables and fruits (organic ones of course!).

- Eat more cruciferous vegetables, like broccoli, brussel sprouts, cabbage and cauliflower, because they are high in a substance called indole-3-carbinol which reduces the metabolism of oestrogen into a toxic form while speeding up its elimination.
- Eat phytoestrogens, like soya, which can reduce the toxic forms of oestrogen in the body.

You may be saying to yourself: 'Why can't they leave our food alone?' Unfortunately, the producers' agenda is never health or safety. It is always financial. But it is important to emphasise that you do have a good deal of control over the food you eat. The British public has been much quicker than the Americans to reject GM foods, forcing the issue out into the open and proving that public pressure does make a difference. For example, in 1989 a chemical called alar that was routinely sprayed on apples was withdrawn after mothers organised a nationwide protest against the suspected cancer-causing chemical. Once you realise what is in the food we eat, you will probably want your family to be protected from the dangers all the time – not just when you are trying to conceive. Get a water filter that can remove a high percentage of oestrogens from the water supply (see Healthy House – in Useful Addresses on page 227). Some filters can also remove pesticide residues, fluoride and heavy metals like lead.

In Your Home

Household pesticides

A number of children have been diagnosed with Charge Syndrome which is characterised by major abnormalities including heart disease. It's believed that the condition is caused by exposure to pesticides and insecticides during pregnancy. One baby was born with severe handicaps after her mother had been exposed to a cockroach pesticide when she was six weeks pregnant. Another woman gave birth to a handicapped child after exposure to flea insecticide during pregnancy.

Dr Jeff Howell, of South Bank University, has strong concerns about the use of permethrin to treat woodworm. This chemical has been linked to skin and eye irritations but also to birth defects. Home-owners have always been told that the treatment chemicals fall to safe levels eight hours after application. But research carried out by the Faunhofer Institute of Toxicology and Aerosol Research in Germany shows that house dust picks up permethrin and deposits it on food and kitchen surfaces. So you can end up breathing and eating it.

Parents in the UK and USA are suing the manufacturers of a garden pesticide they claim caused eye deformities in babies following use in the early months of pregnancy.

What You Can Do

- Try not to use pesticides in your garden. If this is not possible then make sure you don't handle any of this stuff in the four months leading up to conception.
- Do not have your home treated for woodworm in those four months either. Do any house treatments before you actually move in so that you are not living, breathing, eating and sleeping in a potentially toxic environment.
- Treat your pets for fleas with natural herbal sprays. They do not kill the fleas but repel them, making them less likely to stay on the animal. There are also other ways of dealing with fleas which can be obtained from the vet. You can feed your cat a substance or put drops on their necks which changes the blood so the fleas don't like the taste. Garlic works the same way. If you crush up garlic tablets into your pet's feed, this may keep the fleas off.
- Garlic can also be used to deter other insects. A few years ago we had some ants in the kitchen. We opened up some garlic capsules and spread the garlic around the opening the ants seemed to be coming from. Interestingly, the ants would not cross over the 'garlic' line and went back down the crack.

Household Chemicals

Decorating your home can be a problem. Solvent-based paints and white spirits release gases into the air and these can stay around for weeks after painting has finished. Apart from causing irritation, these gases can be inhaled and cause dizziness, nausea and headaches. Years ago, paint and furnishings were made from natural products but nowadays they are usually made from chemicals. Unfortunately, there is also a tendency to paint the baby's room just before it is born so the baby ends up sleeping in a sea of chemicals. In addition, new carpets often contain a chemical preservative called formaldehyde which can irritate the mucus linings of the eyes, nose and throat.

What You Can Do

- Decorate at least four months before conception.
- When you redecorate, buy solvent-free paints.
- Minimise the amount of chemicals you use in your home (such as polish, bleach, detergents, air fresheners, etc). Buy more natural and more biodegradable household cleaners, available from healthfood shops.

Radiation

Our homes are full of devices which emit electromagnetic radiation, including televisions, radios, mobile phones and microwave ovens.

Here are some simple tips to reduce your exposure to radiation at home:

- Don't use an electric blanket which can stay on all night. Apart from the electromagnetic radiation, it can also be too hot for the man's sperm. It is better to heat the bed up first and then switch it off. Better still, use an old-fashioned hot water bottle.
- Position electrical alarm clocks and radios so that they are not right next to your head while you are sleeping.
- Keep a good distance away from televisions and VDUs.

Mobile Phones

To reduce the risk from mobile phones:

- Keep use of your mobile phone down to a minimum and use a landline whenever possible.
- Buy a separate mike so that the handset is not next to your head.
- When the phone is being carried, or if you are using a mike, keep the handset as far away from your body as possible. I regularly see men carrying a mobile phone in their breast pocket right over their heart.

Microwave Ovens

What you can do:

- Think whether you really need to use a microwave oven at all.
- If you continue to cook with a microwave then do not stand directly in front of the oven, especially if you are pregnant.
- Have the oven checked periodically for leaks.
- *Never* open the door when the oven is on.

Lead

In older homes water supplies may contain high levels of lead from lead pipes leading into the house, especially if the water is soft. Even if your pipes are copper (which can carry its own problems), then the pipes may be joined by lead solder, or the pipes to the street may be lead. Lead can leach into the water just by standing in lead pipes overnight so allow the tap to run for a minute first thing in the morning. Always use water from the cold tap, not the hot one, for cooking, making hot drinks, etc, because lead dissolves more easily into hot water.

It is now well-known that lead, especially from petrol fumes, can have a disastrous effect on the behavioural and intellectual development of children.[157]

Leaded petrol has been gradually phased out, with more and more cars running on lead-free petrol. Since January 2000 it has not be available at all.

What You Can Do

- Since the 1960s all paint has been lead-free, but if you are renovating an old house then you must be careful when scraping or burning off old paint. Take extra precautions, such as wearing a mask; and have good ventilation, or get a professional to do the job. Also make sure that enough time is left for the renovations to be completed before the four-month preconception period.
- If at all possible, try to live away from very busy roads where lead levels could be high. Otherwise use net curtains to try to lessen your exposure.
- Use a water filter for all your water, including cooking, hot drinks, etc. Either get a simple jug water filter or a filter that is fitted under the sink that runs into the cold water supply. The choice of a filter is not easy because a jug filter is made of plastic (raising concerns about xenoestrogens) and bottled water often comes in plastic. The experts are now asking to know what the plastics are made from, as not all plastics leach chemicals and then we could make an informed choice.

- If you are unsure about your water supply, or if you have lead pipes or a lead tank, then you can ask your local environmental health department or water supplier to test the water for you. Your public library should have a copy of the *Drinking Water Inspectorate's Annual Report* which details the monitoring of the water supply and when the water has exceeded 'maximum permitted levels'. (A few years ago there was a problem with my local water and the public were told that it was safe to drink but not to use it to fill up fish tanks, as it could kill the fish. That gave everybody confidence!)

Aluminium

Aluminium has been linked to dementia because it has been found in patches of cell damage in the brains of people with Alzheimer's. The results are not conclusive but we should perhaps be wary of it anyway.

The main sources of aluminium are indigestion tablets (antacids), deodorants and anti-perspirants, anti-caking agents found in some dried milk, aluminium cookware, soft drink cans and foil. High levels of aluminium can be seen from the analysis of a hair sample (see page 102).

What You Can Do

- Buy aluminium-free deodorants at healthfood shops, where the ingredients will be listed on the containers.
- If you are taking indigestion tablets, have the cause of the problem investigated either medically or with a good nutritional therapist (see Useful Addresses).
- Get rid of all your aluminium pans and buy cast iron, enamel, glass and stainless steel. (People used to cook rhubarb (a very acidic fruit) in an aluminium pan to 'clean' up the pan, which it did very nicely, as the aluminium was neatly absorbed into the rhubarb.)
- The same applies to acid drinks like colas in aluminium cans. They should be avoided for a number of reasons, including the leaching of aluminium into the drink.

Cadmium

This is an inorganic poison present in tobacco smoke and is a well-known mutagen (see page 75). It interferes with your zinc levels which are crucial for both male and female fertility. The main answer is for both of you to stop smoking.

At Work

You or your partner may be in a job that regularly exposes you to hazards (see Chapter 5) and you will need to think about whether the risk can be minimised or whether you may have to change your occupation.

For example, working with lead (used to make storage batteries), radiation, pesticides and solvents can be a problem. If you work in a dry cleaners or hairdressers you are likely to come into contact with many different chemicals.

Visual Display Units

Research on the risks of radiation from VDUs is still in its early stages. However, you can reduce the risk if you:

- Keep the time spent on the VDU to a minimum, with the most being four hours per day.
- Ask your employer if it's possible to give you other, non-computer work for at least the first three months of pregnancy.
- Use houseplants to stop the air becoming too dry. (Some plants are able to absorb a certain amount of radiation and to act as air purifiers, according to a NASA space project, which showed that the plants could remove toxic substances like carbon monoxide from the air. The most beneficial plants are the tropical ones such as lady palm (*Rhapis*), bamboo, parlour palm (*Chaemaedorea*), ficus, peace lily (*Spathiphyllum*) and spider plants.)

Occupational Hazards for Your Partner

The male organs are on the outside of the body for a good reason. The testes need to be several degrees cooler than body temperature because sperm production can only take place at 32°C (89°F). And our normal body temperature is 37°C (98.4°F). Anything that brings the testes closer to the body, and so raises their temperature, may affect the sperm count. An increased temperature of only 1°C has been shown to decrease the sperm count by about 14 per cent.[158]

A number of studies on drivers have found that men who spend more than three hours a day in a car or lorry are less fertile.[159] When men drive they are not only sitting for a long time but are getting the vibrations from the vehicle. So they are literally 'in the hot seat'.

The same research showed that men who are exposed to heat during their work are four times less likely to make their partner pregnant within three months. This might apply to a range of occupations – including anyone working with boilers or welding. One man I saw, who is a baker, was getting great blasts of heat directly on his genital area every time he opened an oven door.

What He Can Do

- Avoid crossing his legs when sitting down.
- Take regular breaks to move around.
- Avoid wearing tight trousers or underpants which constrict the testes.
- Avoid hot baths – he should shower instead.
- Shower his genitals with cold water to lower their temperature and improve circulation.
- Avoid using electric blankets – particularly once he is in bed.

Exercise

It is important to have a good level of physical activity because it improves heart function, controls cholesterol, reduces blood pressure, reduces excess weight and generally optimises health. But it is also important to keep a balance and some sports may compromise male fertility.

If a man exercises excessively it can lower his sperm count. Long hours of training for a marathon, for instance, could therefore be a problem.

Very vigorous sports, like squash or running, may not be advisable because of the knocking effect of the testes against the thighs as the man runs.

Likewise tight-fitting nylon shorts, either worn on their own for running or under shorts in the gym, may contribute to male fertility problems.

Finally, men who regularly go for long bike trips, especially on a racing bike, may spend a lot of time bent over, bringing the testes quite close to the body and crushing them against the seat of the bike, causing overheating and constriction.

Going To The Dentist

Dental work is a major source of mercury pollution. So you need to find a dentist who specialises in mercury-free dentistry.

He or she can test whether any mercury vapour is leaking from your fillings. Any excess mercury will also show up in the hair analysis (see page 102). If there are no signs that mercury is leaking from fillings then it is better to leave well alone. Digging up old fillings can release mercury that was in fact dormant. If fillings have to be removed there are ways to minimise the release and absorption of this old mercury. If new fillings are needed then ask for alternatives to amalgam. You don't want a new filling releasing mercury while you are trying to conceive.

You will probably have to pay for the alternative fillings, as they are not likely to be covered on the NHS.

My advice is that you should have any necessary dental work done at the beginning of the Four-Month Preconception Plan and avoid any dental X-rays, fillings and anaesthetic, once you are trying to conceive. You will be two weeks pregnant before you know you are and it is best to avoid any dental work once you are pregnant, unless it is an emergency.

CHAPTER 14

Overcoming Medical Problems

You may have been told that there is a specific recognised medical problem that is preventing you and your partner conceiving – probably one of the conditions listed in Chapter 3. You must not lose heart if this is the case. Not only can these conditions be eased by a general improvement in your health but there are also natural remedies that can help overcome them, even when conventional medicine has failed.

Female Medical Problems

Coeliac Disease

This digestive disorder, which is not just a female disorder, is an intolerance to gluten which is found in grains such as wheat, rye, barley and oats. Before diagnosis the intolerance causes malabsorption and can therefore leave you deficient in vital nutrients. Many deficiencies have been noted in sufferers of coeliac disease, including folic acid, vitamins A, D, E, K and the B vitamins, zinc (essential for fertility) and selenium.[160] It is known that women with coeliac disease can be subfertile and this is yet another indication that having the correct levels of vitamins and minerals can play an important role in increasing fertility.

Natural Treatment

If you have been diagnosed with coeliac disease you first need to remove gluten from your diet. You will probably have been given dietary advice with the diagnosis which means that you will have to eliminate wheat, rye, barley and oats and substitute other foods like rice cakes, gluten-free bread and also pasta made without gluten such as corn and millet pastas. Then you need a nutritional assessment (see Useful Addresses) to ascertain which supplements are required to correct any deficiencies. Remember that any food supplements (e.g. multivitamin and mineral for pregnancy) must be gluten-free.

Polycystic Ovary Syndrome

There is a difference between having polycystic ovaries and having polycystic ovary syndrome. When ovaries are seen on an ultrasound scan, they can look polycystic, which means that a number of partially developed follicles can be seen. Of course, follicles have to be present for eggs to develop adequately, and so that ovulation can occur. However, with polycystic ovaries, the ovaries are larger than normal and the undeveloped follicles resemble a bunch of grapes. This is very common and does not necessarily present a problem. It is only when the polycystic ovaries lead to a hormonal imbalance that a woman is said to have polycystic ovary syndrome (PCOS) where she will probably not be ovulating and can be overweight and have excess body hair, skin problems and mood swings. The hormone imbalance is produced by having high levels of LH (luteinising hormone) and a higher than normal level of free testosterone, particularly in overweight sufferers.

Just before ovulation in a normal menstrual cycle, LH levels rise dramatically. This is called the LH surge and causes an egg to be released from a follicle. If LH is high during the whole of the follicular phase (the phase before ovulation), then the LH surge does not take place and an egg is not released. High levels of LH have been implicated in both infertility and miscarriage.[161] Doctors have not yet found out why high levels of LH may cause infertility or miscarriage, but research is continuing.

In summary, a woman with PCOS can have:

- high levels of LH
- high oestrogen
- higher than normal male hormones (androgens)
- low progesterone

Diagnosis

This is usually made by ultrasound or a laparoscopy, where a narrow tube with a telescopic lens is inserted into the abdomen via a small incision below the navel. These investigations are conducted together with hormone blood tests.

Medical Treatments

If you are trying to conceive it is imperative that you start to ovulate. One of the most common drugs used to trigger ovulation is clomiphene citrate. Clomiphene is an anti-oestrogen that tricks the brain into thinking that there is no oestrogen in the blood. Because the oestrogen is blocked, the pituitary gland gets the message to increase the supply of follicle stimulating hormone (FSH). The FSH reaches the ovaries and egg production is stimulated. If the clomiphene is suddenly stopped, the brain recognises that there is a massive amount of oestrogen and this results in an LH surge that releases the egg from the ovary.

Clomiphene is an effective drug for artificially inducing ovulation but, ironically, it may also increase the chances of a miscarriage by somewhere in the region of 20–30 per cent.[162] It is thought that the clomiphene interferes with the womb lining, preventing the fertilised egg from implanting. Other treatments used to induce ovulation, like gonadotrophin treatment, can also increase the miscarriage rate.

Natural Treatment

Losing weight has been shown to be very effective in treating PCOS and restoring fertility. One study showed that overweight women with PCOS had more fertility problems than lean women with PCOS.[163] However, even though the link between PCOS and excess weight (and between losing weight and reduced symptoms) is well-established, the reasons for it are unclear.

Nevertheless, overweight women seem to have much lower levels of sex hormone binding globulin (SHBG) in their blood which resulted in more testosterone and worse PCOS symptoms, such as an excess of hair.

When these women went on a diet and lost weight their SHBG levels rose, their testosterone levels fell and their PCOS symptoms diminished.[164]

Along with the weight loss came a remarkable change in ovarian function: 82 per cent of the women who were not previously ovulating showed improvements, with a number of successful pregnancies occurring during the study, even though these women had a long-standing history of infertility.[165]

One reason may be that weight loss lowers insulin levels, which reduces the ovaries' production of testosterone. No one really knows why PCOS responds to weight loss but it must be linked with the fact that overweight women (without PCOS) can dramatically increase their fertility by losing weight.

One study found that 11 out of 12 women who had been overweight and not ovulating conceived naturally after reducing weight.[165]

For more on natural treatment of PCOS, see page 125.

Fibroids

Fibroids, which are non-cancerous growths, are given different names depending on where they grow:

- **Submucosal fibroids** grow on the inside of the womb and extend into the uterine cavity.

- **Intramural fibroids** grow within the uterine wall.

- **Subserol fibroids** grow on the outside of the womb, in the lining between the uterus and the pelvic cavity.

The main symptoms of fibroids is extremely heavy periods. If the fibroid is submucosal, then the mechanism that stops menstrual flow may not operate effectively. Menstrual flow is stopped by muscular contractions of the womb and fibroids can interfere with this.

Diagnosis

Fibroids can be diagnosed in several ways. Often they are picked up on a simple internal examination. If the fibroids are small, then a pelvic ultrasound can be used and this is often done to confirm the diagnosis from the internal examination.

Medical Treatment

If the fibroids are preventing pregnancy and they are not too large, they can be removed surgically, leaving the womb intact (myomectomy).

Recently, a new technique has been developed called arterial embolisation. Fibroids have their own blood supply and the theory is that, if that blood supply is cut off, the fibroids will stop growing and may even shrink. Embolisation is performed with a laser and it can make some fibroids shrink to one-third of their original size.

Natural Treatment

The natural treatment for fibroids is the same as that for PCOS and endometriosis (see page 125).

Endometriosis

Endometriosis occurs when the lining of the womb starts growing in other places in the body. It can cause extremely painful periods and also painful sex. Yet some women have endometriosis and experience no symptoms at all.

Diagnosis

Diagnosis is by laparoscopy. It is performed under a general anaesthetic and allows a good view of the womb, fallopian tubes and ovaries.

WHAT CAUSES ENDOMETRIOSIS?

There is some disagreement on this among the medical profession. Some suggest that endometriosis is due to migration of the endometrial tissue up the fallopian tubes and into the abdomen. The flaw in this theory is that some women who have been sterilised (i.e. had their fallopian tubes tied or cut) still get endometriosis. The other possibility is that it happens during foetal development when young endometrial cells are displaced and then only begin to grow when the girl reaches puberty. This might explain why endometriosis appears to run in families.

Medical Treatments

Spots of endometriosis can be burned off with diathermy (the use of intense heat) or laser. If a large chocolate (blood-filled) cyst has taken over the ovary, then the surgeon uses the laser to open up the cyst to allow the old blood to drain out. Surgery presents a risk of scar tissue being created so it is kept to a minimum.

Because endometriosis is influenced by the menstrual cycle, drug treatment involves shutting down the female hormone pattern so that periods do not occur. Like fibroids, endometriosis is oestrogen-dependent, so the aim is to reduce the amount of oestrogen in the body. The contraceptive pill has been used to treat endometriosis but, in order for the treatment to be effective, all breakthrough bleeding must stop. This usually requires high-dosage pills which can have unpleasant side-effects.

The main drug treatment for endometriosis is danazol. This is a synthetic weak male hormone that stops ovulation. This, in turn, stops the womb lining from developing. Again, like most drugs, it has side-effects, which some women can tolerate and others can't. The side-effects can include severe mood swings, nausea, dizziness, rashes and headaches. Because dana-zol is a mild male hormone, additional side-effects may include facial hair, acne, increased sex drive and weight gain.

Recent advances have produced new drugs that contain gonadotrophin-releasing hormone (GnRH). This drug produces a temporary menopause and the endometriosis shrinks. The most common one used is goserelin which has to be given by injection. Because the woman goes through a temporary menopause, one of the major symptoms is hot flushes.

Natural Treatments for PCOS, Fibroids and Endometriosis

Although polycystic ovary syndrome, fibroids and endometriosis are differ-ent conditions, they can often be triggered by the same mechanisms – hor-mone imbalances, stress and nutritional deficiencies. By getting back into optimum health, it is often possible to alleviate or eliminate these problems.

All three conditions are connected to oestrogen: both fibroids and endometriosis are sensitive to oestrogen and PCOS is characterised by high levels of oestrogen as well as other hormones like LH. When you are over-weight, you have more circulating oestrogen because it is produced by fat cells. So, with any of these problems, it is important to lose any excess weight.

For all these conditions, it is also important that your liver is functioning well. The liver is the body's waste disposal unit, not only for toxins and waste products but also for hormones. If your liver is not functioning effi-ciently, you may therefore get an accumulation of 'old' hormones left over from each menstrual cycle. The liver deactivates these 'old' hormones and renders them harmless. The B vitamins are essential for the liver to be able to carry out this conversion.

With PCOS, you need to lose weight in order to correct the underlying problem so that you begin to ovulate on your own. If you are just given clomiphene to make you ovulate, when you stop taking the clomiphene you are in exactly the same situation as when you started. Similarly, the aim of the natural approach for fibroids and endometriosis is to address the underlying cause of the problem rather than the symptoms.

Dietary measures

By making the following dietary changes, you can positively affect the under-lying cause of PCOS, fibroids or endometriosis and so aid your fertility:

- **Reduce your saturated fat intake.** A diet high in the saturated fat found in red meat is known to stimulate oestrogen over-production, so a diet free of animal products (except fish) could help.[167] If you still have a high intake of saturated fats, taking *Lactobacillus acidophilus* as a supplement seems to help because it lowers the level of the enzymes which reabsorb the 'old' hormones.

  The saturated fats in red meat and poultry produce hormones called prostaglandins. The particular prostaglandin produced from saturated fats is highly inflammatory and can cause swelling and pain. This hormone can trigger muscle contraction and constriction in the blood vessels, so it can worsen period pains, endometriosis-related cramps and the spread of endometrial tissue.

- **Increase your fibre intake.** The amount of fibre in your diet is important too because the fibre contained in grains and vegetables reduces oestrogen levels and seems to work by 'shielding' oestrogens that are excreted in the bile, so preventing them from being reabsorbed back into the blood. Women who eat a vegetarian diet excrete three times more 'old', detoxified oestrogens than women who eat meat. The meat-eaters also reabsorb more oestrogen.

- **Reduce or eliminate sugar.** Sugar is bad for PCOS, fibroids and endometriosis because it increases fat, which then increases oestrogen production. Sugar also depletes the body of valuable nutrients.

- **Reduce or eliminate caffeine.** Caffeine has a diuretic effect and so depletes valuable stores of vitamins and minerals that are essential for a healthy hormone balance. Also, drinking more than two cups of coffee a day has been linked to endometriosis and tubal damage.[168]

  The effects of caffeine and its links to miscarriage are discussed in detail in Section 5.

• **Eliminate alcohol.** If you are trying to conceive, you need to eliminate alcohol (see Chapters 2 and 8). It should also be eliminated to help conditions such as PCOS, fibroids and endometriosis. Like dairy products and saturated fats, alcohol can compromise the efficient functioning of the liver and make it less able to metabolise hormones.

Alcohol is a good example of a substance that damages us by interfering with the positive action of nutrients and affecting their absorption. As such, it is classed as an anti-nutrient because it depletes the body of vitamin B6, iron and zinc.

Exercise

Exercise is also highly beneficial, as it can help alleviate period pains by increasing circulation to the pelvic region. Exercise can also reduce stress and it is well known that exercise releases brain chemicals called endorphins which make us feel calmer, happier and more alert.

Exercise alone has been shown to have a very positive effect on people suffering from depression, stress, anxiety and insomnia and it is now often recommended as part of the treatment for these problems. Stress can have a direct effect on fertility so it is important to find ways of dealing with it.

Exercise can also have a direct effect on controlling oestrogen. A fascinating study, reported in the *US Journal of the National Cancer Institute*, showed that women who exercised for around four hours a week had a 58 per cent lower risk of breast cancer and those who routinely exercised for between one and three hours a week had a 30 per cent lower risk.[169] Regular exercise seems to modify a woman's hormonal activity in a beneficial way. We know that extremes of exercise alter the menstrual cycle dramatically – many women athletes, for instance, don't have periods at all. So moderate routine exercise may suppress the production (or over-production) of hormones, reducing a woman's exposure during her lifetime. Some breast cancers are oestrogen-sensitive so it makes sense that if the hormone levels are more balanced then the risk of developing breast cancer will be lower. This knowledge is also valuable in other conditions where excess oestrogen may be a problem (e.g. PCOS, fibroids and endometriosis).

Herbs

Herbs can have a tremendous impact on these three conditions. If your problem is long-standing, it may be worth asking a medical herbalist for a private consultation (see Useful Addresses).

- **Agnus castus** (vitex/chasteberry) is one of the most important herbs for female hormone problems. It stimulates and normalises the function of the pituitary gland, which controls and balances the hormones in the body. Agnus castus works by restoring the balance, whether it is a hormone deficit or an excess.

- **Milk thistle** is an excellent herb for the liver and a number of studies have shown that its use can result in an increase of new liver cells to replace old damaged ones.[170] Silymarin is the collective name for the substances found in milk thistle that produce this beneficial effect.

- **Dandelion** also helps cleanse the liver, the major organ of detoxification, which gets rid of accumulated 'old' female hormones.

Essential fatty acids

Our bodies produce beneficial prostaglandins from essential fatty acids. These prostaglandins help reduce period pains and they also have an anti-inflammatory effect which is especially beneficial for endometriosis sufferers.

Zinc and vitamin B6 are also important for the correct metabolism of fatty acids and their conversion to beneficial prostaglandins (PGE1 and PGE3). However, certain prostaglandins (PGE2) can have a negative effect in large amounts. They are highly inflammatory, and can cause swelling and pain and also thicken the blood.

In a 1998 study, women with endometriosis were asked to eliminate caffeine, to control blood sugar (and the over-excretion of insulin), and to supplement with essential fatty acids. The doctors found that by making these simple dietary changes, the women experienced a significant decrease in their symptoms.[171] The control of blood sugar is also central to the dietary treatment of PCOS.

Summary

To ease fertility problems naturally, you need to:

- eliminate caffeine
- reduce or eliminate saturated fats
- eliminate alcohol
- get your weight within a BMI of 20–24 (see page 58)

SECTION 3

SEEKING MEDICAL
HELP

❖

Having read Sections 1 and 2, you are probably beginning to understand how the complex and delicate balance of our reproductive systems can be upset by things we do, eat, or come into contact with in everyday life. Of all these factors, nutrition (getting your diet right and correcting any deficiencies) is probably the most important. It's certainly a vital first step for any couple trying to improve their fertility, even if they eventually opt for an assisted conception.

However, when you keep trying to conceive and nothing happens it is easy to get into a panic and start thinking that something is seriously wrong – either with you or your partner. So in this section I describe the various medical tests you can both have, in order to check different aspects of your fertility. These tests can highlight specific medical problems and assess crucial factors like hormone levels and sperm quality. Sometimes simply going through the process of eliminating different possibilities can give you peace of mind and make you more relaxed (which can be helpful in itself). And the information you gain may be very useful. For instance, if you find that your partner has poor sperm motility you can target the problem directly with additional nutrients like L-arginine (see page 91).

The table below gives a summary of the different causes of infertility in Britain. As you can see, the largest percentage of infertility (30 per cent) is 'unexplained'. This means the doctors have investigated the couple but that no specific medical problem can be identified. It also underlines my point – that lifestyle and environmental factors can play a vital role in fertility problems and they usually require self-help strategies rather than medical intervention.

CAUSES OF INFERTILITY IN BRITAIN

Ovulatory failure (including PCOS)	20%
Tubal damage	15%
Endometriosis	5%
Male problems	40%
Unexplained	30%

The total comes to more than 100 per cent because some couples' infertility can have more than one cause.

Case History

Barbara was 41 when she came to see me. She had tried four IUI cycles with no success. She had been told her FSH levels were too high, ranging from 24 to 33 at the beginning of her cycles over a number of months. The cut-off level is 10 for most IVF clinics and levels as high as Barbara's would normally indicate that she was beginning the menopause. The clinic had asked her to be tested each month to see how the FSH was fluctuating. Although the clinic was focusing on Barbara's hormone levels, I still suggested that both she and her partner should be tested for nutritional deficiencies and have these corrected, which they did. They both followed the Four-Month Preconception Plan outlined in this book and Barbara conceived naturally on a cycle with an FSH of 24. She now has a healthy baby boy.

Although it is important to investigate any possible medical problems, most couples are better advised only to start these investigations once they have implemented their preconception dietary and lifestyle changes by following the four-month plan. They should then try to conceive on their own for approximately six months. This is because many of the factors that will be tested – such as hormone levels, ovulation and sperm quality – will start to improve very quickly of their own accord, once both partners have established the recommended changes. The only exceptions to this are couples where the woman is older than 35 or couples who have reason to believe that they have a medical problem (such as the symptoms of an infection, which should be treated immediately).

CHAPTER 15

Identifying the Problem

It is now taking young couples, on average, up to three years to conceive. So if you are young (20–30 years), with no known problems, you should really wait for 12 months before approaching your doctor for help.

However, if you are over 35 you should go and see your doctor if you have not conceived after six months. Biologically it is just that much harder for you to conceive and you do not, at your age, have that much time to wait.

Blood Tests

Usually your GP will offer you a blood test to measure your progesterone levels. This '21-day' test is done seven days after ovulation (14 days from the start of the period to ovulation, plus seven days after that) and can indicate if you have actually ovulated.

If the blood test is normal you will probably be told to keep trying for a while. If the blood test shows low progesterone or some other problem you will probably be referred to a gynaecologist.

Make sure the doctor knows if you have an irregular cycle. Otherwise the 21-day progesterone blood test may be done on the wrong day and give the wrong information. For example, if you have a 35-day cycle then you could be ovulating on approximately day 18 of the cycle. So, if you are tested on day 21, it would look as if your progesterone was low when in fact you were only three days after ovulation instead of seven.

> **WARNING**
>
> Traditionally, drugs like clomiphene citrate (which induce ovulation) are prescribed, sometimes without any tests, if a woman is not conceiving. But these drugs are only helpful if you are not ovulating. Many women have been given the drug and found out later that they were ovulating anyway and their problem was due to something else.

Other Tests

The gynaecologist may suggest other tests such as:

- **A laparoscopy**, a diagnostic procedure whereby a laparoscope (a narrow instrument with a telescopic lens) is inserted via a small incision below the navel to see the uterus, fallopian tubes, ovaries and other abdominal organs.

- **A hysterosalpingogram (HSG)**, an X-ray procedure in which a special opaque dye is injected through the cervix to see the inside of the uterus and the openness (patency) of the fallopian tubes. This should be done in the first half of the menstrual cycle in case you are already pregnant.

- **A hysterosalpingosonogram (HSS)**, which is similar to HSG above but uses ultrasound instead of X-rays to assess the tubes. It is also very valuable for examining the uterine cavity.

- **A hysteroscopy**, a diagnostic procedure in which a hysteroscope (a lighted scope) is inserted through the cervix in order to view the inside of the uterus.

How Long do the Tests Take?

There are often waiting lists for these tests and the National Health Service, with the best will in the world, is under time pressures and financial constraints which slow the process down. Time is spent waiting for the next consultation and months pass. For some couples I've seen it's taken upwards of three years to have a full set of investigations and they were still unsure of the findings. Unfortunately, with each passing year the woman is getting older and, by implication, her fertility is decreasing. With many women following careers in the early part of their lives and delaying pregnancy until later, they may not find out that they have any fertility problems until well into their thirties, so time is of the essence.

Is There an Alternative?

To shorten this process, pioneering work has been carried out by a number of doctors to help couples get more definite answers more quickly. One clinic, Reproductive Healthcare in North London (see Useful Addresses), uses a process called a monitored cycle. This involves taking a number of 'snapshot' tests over one menstrual cycle to identify the particular point where the cycle is not functioning. Conventionally, tests are all done on different cycles, a 21-day blood test in one month, maybe a laparoscopy another month. But doing it this way makes it hard to get the 'big picture' about what is actually happening with your reproductive system. You get more complete information by closely monitoring a single menstrual cycle. The monitored cycle looks at hormonal balance and reproductive function and the way they work together.

Monitored Cycle Using Ultrasound and Blood Tests

At the beginning of the cycle, between days 1 and 3, a blood test is taken to measure oestradiol (from the ovary) and LH and FSH (from the pituitary gland) and to check the egg reserve. This blood test is very useful for older women as it can give an indication of the likelihood of conceiving (ovarian reserve). The blood test also checks the hormone output from the thyroid gland as well as prolactin, both of which are essential for normal fertility function.

The first ultrasound scan is done between days 6 and 8 of the cycle (day 1 is the first day of the period).

Approximately three serial scans are performed during the cycle. These can show the thickness of the womb lining, and the size, growth and blood flow to the developing follicle in the ovary.

A scan a week after ovulation checks on the functioning of the corpus luteum (which pumps out progesterone, the hormone needed to maintain a pregnancy). The scan at this stage can also determine whether the womb lining is thick enough for a fertilised embryo to be implanted.

A blood test is also performed after ovulation to check on the hormone progesterone.

There is also a test called a hysterosalpingosonogram (HSS) which is usually performed before ovulation to check that there are no blockages in your fallopian tubes. This is an alternative to HSG (see page 132) because it can be done in the first part of the cycle which means that the gynaecologist can have a complete set of information by the end of that particular cycle. The HSS does not involve the use of X-rays so there is no radiation risk. A sterile fluid is injected into the uterus and traced with ultrasound as it passes through the fallopian tubes. The scan outlines the uterine cavity and the tubes and shows the spill of fluid around the ovaries.

You can get these monitored cycle investigations done through the NHS. Ask your gynaecologist about it. Otherwise you may need to find a private hospital unit or clinic that offers this approach.

Monitored Cycle Using Saliva

This is a very simple test which is done at home and sent to the lab for analysis. A total of 11 saliva samples are collected over one cycle at specific times. The level of the hormones oestrogen and progesterone are mapped for that month to provide a pattern which can reveal:

• early ovulation
• anovulation (no ovulation)
• problems with the phasing of the cycle, such as a short luteal phase (second half of cycle)
• problems with maintaining progesterone levels

This test can still be done even if you have irregular cycles and the graph opposite shows an actual cycle taken from a patient.

This patient (aged 34) was having trouble conceiving and was also having breakthrough bleeding for a few days before each period started.

Her cycle was 26 days but she was ovulating around day 17 which meant that there were just nine days between ovulation and her period. This is called a luteal phase defect (when the length of the second half of the cycle is less than 12 days).

The graph shows that the patient's progesterone output was almost finished by day 21 which meant that it only stayed high for four days after ovulation.

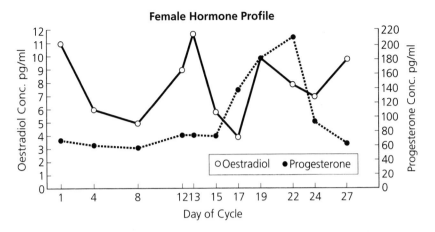

Female Hormone Profile

Oestradiol Conc. pg/ml

Progesterone Conc. pg/ml

Day of Cycle

○ Oestradiol ● Progesterone

Sample Cycle Mapping Levels of Hormones Using Saliva

The breakthrough bleeding was explained by the early drop in progesterone levels. With progesterone output like this, a patient could conceive but would find it hard to maintain a pregnancy. The chances are she would not even know that she was pregnant.

Depending on the problems found, it may be possible to correct hormone irregularities with nutritional supplements or herbs. The patient can then do another test in three months to confirm whether this has helped. If the problem looks very severe or if the patient is over 35 it is worth starting further investigations right away.

Which Monitored Cycle to Choose?

The monitored cycle using ultrasound and blood tests gives extra information, in that the development and thickness of the womb lining can be assessed at the same time as looking at hormone balance.

However the saliva monitored cycle is *very* convenient as a first step because you don't need to go into a clinic during the cycle. You can take the samples at home and have the kit sent by post through me or another competent practitioner (see page 227).

CHAPTER 16

The Man's Role

Up to 40 per cent of infertility problems can be on the man's side and yet the focus, particularly in the early stages of investigation, is usually on the woman. Until recently, the only investigation available for a partner was a basic analysis of a semen sample.

Infertility consultations should include both partners. But most infertility clinics are run by gynaecologists who are specialists in the female reproductive system and regard the man as a bit of an afterthought. I find women often come to me on their own because their partners say 'it's not my problem'. Men emotionally connect virility with fertility and feel somehow 'less of a man' if they are not able to give their partner a child. Women seem to be able to distance their emotions a little better from problems with their reproductive system. But 'it takes two to tango', as the saying goes, and your partner needs to remember that he is contributing 50 per cent not only to the health of the baby but also to you getting pregnant in the first place.

Your partner should therefore be involved in investigations from the beginning. You may, for example, have a situation where you are both sub-fertile and it is this combination that is causing the problem. If you both had different partners, whose fertility was optimum, you could probably conceive fairly easily. By boosting both your levels of fertility you will have a much better chance of conceiving.

The traditional approach – concentrating on investigating your fertility and ignoring your partner – has some unfortunate consequences. If your partner's semen analysis is poor, for instance, you may be advised to go straight for fertility treatments (see Section 4) without any further investigations, even if you yourself may not actually have trouble conceiving. Both IVF and ICSI treatments require you to take large quantities of drugs, while your partner just provides the sperm sample. So, in effect, you would end up being treated when you do not need to be, because there is a problem on your partner's side. This is obviously not very desirable and your partner should have more investigations before you decide to embark on what can be long and stressful fertility treatments.

Some enlightened doctors will refer the man to a urologist who specialises in diseases of the urinary system, including the bladder and kidneys. Urologists treat both men and women. And there are a few andrologists who specialise in problems with the male reproductive system.

Even if the problem initially seems to be on your side it could just mask the real cause. Many women who suffer miscarriages, for instance, assume there is a problem with their own reproductive system. But it is logical that, if there is something wrong with the sperm that fertilises the egg, nature will cause a miscarriage. Studies have shown that there is an increased risk of miscarriage when there are sperm abnormalities.[172] This is why it is so important for *both* of you to get yourselves into optimum health before conception.

Sperm Production

Sperm are manufactured in seminiferous tubules (thread-like structures which fill the two testes). It takes at least three months for sperm cells to mature, ready to be ejaculated. That is why it is vital for a preconception programme to be put into place at least three months (preferably four) before trying to conceive. It is also important that, if there are problems with the sperm (e.g. low motility), then the man should follow a preconception programme for at least three months before re-testing because the benefits may not be apparent before then.

The head of the tadpole-like sperm carries the genetic material which will enter the egg and join the female genetic material. The head of the sperm has to be hard enough and contain certain enzymes in order to penetrate the egg. I have seen a number of couples where the man's semen analysis was fine and there were no problems with his partner. They had been referred for IVF treatment and at the vital point when the egg and sperm were put in the same dish, no fertilisation took place. This highlights an important limitation of semen analysis. It cannot identify one important reason for failure to conceive – the fact that a partner's sperm, however fertile it is, cannot get into the egg.

Sometimes sperm heads are not strong enough to penetrate the egg. Sometimes the egg's outer layer, the zona pellucida, is too tough to be penetrated. Or it could be a combination of both that is making fertilisation difficult.

In this situation, even though the man has a good semen count, you would probably be advised to have ICSI treatment which involves inserting the sperm directly into the egg (see page 168) and is usually used to treat men with extremely low sperm counts. However, it's certainly preferable to try other more natural ways of toughening up the sperm head and increasing the chances of conception before contemplating ICSI.

The middle part of the sperm provides the energy needed by the tail to move forward and also contains the mitochondrial DNA which plays a part in the inheritance of genes.

Also inside the testes are the Leydig cells which produce the hormone testosterone. Like oestrogen in the woman, this hormone is responsible for changes that occur around puberty, resulting in body and facial hair and a deep voice. Testosterone is needed for the sex drive and helping to achieve and maintain an erection.

As in a woman, the pituitary gland plays a large part in fertility because it releases the two vital hormones, follicle stimulating hormone (FSH) and luteinising hormone (LH). It is interesting that we tend to think of 'male' and 'female' hormones and yet both men and women share the same reproductive hormones. The only difference is the proportions of these hormones. Testosterone is often classed as the 'male hormone' and yet women also produce testosterone, which is needed for sex drive just as in the man. However, the ratio of testosterone to oestrogen will be different in the man and the woman, resulting in either female or male characteristics, depending on the dominance of one or other of those hormones.

So we come back again to the idea of balancing our hormones, so that they can function efficiently, in the right amounts, and do the job they are supposed to do. This can be achieved by aiming for optimum health through changes in lifestyle and diet, so that the body has the tools to balance itself – so simple really and yet so effective.

Both women and men produce FSH and LH. In the man FSH is responsible for stimulating the cells in the seminiferous tubules to produce sperm, and LH stimulates the Leydig cells to produce testosterone.

Semen Analysis

This is the most basic male fertility test. The man is asked to produce a sample by masturbating directly into a sterile container. Some clinics will ask the man to collect the sample at home and bring it into the lab within one hour, while others will ask the man to produce the sample at the clinic. The man will be asked to abstain from sex for a minimum of 48 hours but not longer than seven days before giving the sample. Some men may have difficulty producing a sample by masturbation or their personal beliefs may prohibit this. If so, special condoms can be provided by the clinic to collect the sperm. Ordinary condoms cannot be used because lubricants, spermicides and even the type of rubber can affect the sperm.

The lab will look at the sample and measure the following factors:

- the number of sperm per millilitre (i.e. the sperm count)
- the percentage of sperm moving (i.e. motile sperm)
- the quality of that movement called progression (graded from 1–4, with 1 being the highest grade)
- the percentage of abnormal sperm
- volume of semen

The World Health Organisation's 1992 recommendations state that there should be more than 20 million sperm, more than 30 per cent of which should be normal and more than 50 per cent moving actively.

If the woman is fertile then it is still possible for her to conceive with a man whose sperm count is as low as 20 million, as long as everything else about the sperm is healthy.

The medical terms used with the sperm count are oligozoospermia (too few sperm) and azoospermia (no sperm at all). With both of these, further tests should be done to see if there is a reason for the result (see tests below). High levels of abnormal sperm are called teratozoospermia and low motility is called astenozoospermia.

Seminal Volume

The normal volume of seminal fluid is between 2 and 6ml and this level can vary depending on the length of abstinence before giving the sample. If the volume is low, this may interfere with the transportation of the sperm and they may not reach the cervix. If the man has a low volume of semen then the fructose test (see below) is done. This test can show whether there is a blockage in the ducts.

High volume can also be a problem, although this is more unusual. The high volume may dilute the density of the sperm and affect their motion.

As always, it comes back to getting the right balance. It is no good having too few or too many sperm; it can also be a problem if there is too low or too high a volume of semen. The aim is homeostasis, where the body and all its physiological processes are able to maintain their own equilibrium.

If one semen analysis shows up a problem in any area (such as count or motility) it is worth repeating the analysis. Periods of stress, or illnesses such as flu, can produce unusual sperm samples. One man, who had been following the suggestions in this book to improve his sperm sample, re-did the sperm analysis soon after attending his mother's funeral and it looked as if the sperm quality had actually decreased from his previous sample, but the lab rechecked a few weeks later and everything was fine.

Why Are So Many Sperm Needed?

The count is a measurement of how many sperm there are per millilitre, there should be at least 20 million. And yet a man might have a volume of 4ml, which would equal 80 million sperm in that one sample. As it only takes one sperm to fertilise the egg, and indeed nature tries to prevent any other sperm entering once one has penetrated the inner surface, why are millions produced in each ejaculate? As with other aspects of nature, abundance is the rule. Many more seeds are produced from a plant than will actually get a chance to germinate. It is the same with frog spawn where, from that enormous mass, hundreds of tadpoles can emerge but only a small proportion will eventually become frogs. Nature always works on the principle of 'survival of the fittest', basing her calculations on the fact that, from the huge number produced, be it seeds or sperm, many are going to die off en route.

It is estimated that only a small fraction of sperm will actually reach the egg (as few as 100), as the sperm need to swim up the vagina, through the cervix and up the fallopian tubes. Normally only one egg is released and this egg will travel down one fallopian tube, so half of the sperm that are left after the long journey could be travelling up a tube with no egg in it.

When they finally meet the egg, a number of sperm will surround it. On the front of the sperm's head is the acrosomal head cap which contains certain degradative enzymes to help dissolve the cumulous cells surrounding the egg. The combined action of a number of sperm helps with this dissolving process but only one sperm actually gets through the next layer, the zona pellucida. As soon as the egg is penetrated, rapid changes take place in its outer layer and no other sperm can get through.

INTRIGUING FACTS ABOUT SPERM

- A sperm lashes its tail 800 times to travel 1 millimetre.
- Sperm reach the woman's fallopian tubes 30–60 minutes after ejaculation.
- Sperm are produced at an average of 1,500 per second from each testicle.
- In the right conditions, sperm can live up to five days.
- One sperm can swim 3 millimetres per second.

Other Tests

Fructose Test

If there are no sperm in the semen analysis it may mean that none are being produced by the testes, or that they are being produced but the tubes are blocked and they cannot get through to be ejaculated. Where no sperm are present, a test for fructose is done. Fructose is a sugar normally found in semen. The absence of fructose in the semen can mean that the seminal vesicles are blocked, stopping both sperm and fructose from getting through. It may be possible to surgically correct such a blockage. Alternatively, the absence of fructose could mean that the man does not have any seminal vesicles.

If fructose is present but the man does not have any sperm in the sample, further investigations need to be done. These can reveal whether there is a blockage nearer to the testes or whether the testes are not in fact producing sperm.

Anti-sperm Antibody Test

This test attempts to determine whether the man is producing substances which are causing the sperm to clump together, lose motility or prevent fertilisation. These antibodies would make the man's immune system 'see' his own sperm as foreign bodies and try to destroy them.

The most common test for antibodies is the MAR (mixed antiglobulin reaction) test which is now often done as part of the normal semen analysis. If antibodies are present, the sperm will be clumped together instead of moving freely.

Sperm antibodies can be produced in response to an infection. Antibodies can also be produced in about 70 per cent of men after a vasectomy. During the procedure some sperm may leak out and, because previously they had been contained within the reproductive system, the body views them as a foreign substance and produces antibodies to them.

Treatments for anti-sperm antibodies may include steroids which carry their own side-effects, such as weight gain, stomach bleeding and depression. IVF may be a possibility if the sperm can still penetrate the egg, otherwise ICSI will be suggested (see Chapter 19).

It is also possible for the woman to be producing antibodies to her partner's sperm and this can be checked by a blood test.

Post-coital Test

The post-coital test has been used since the 1860s to assess the cervical mucus and the sperm's ability to swim through it. You go to the clinic around the time of ovulation after having intercourse about four to ten hours before. A cervical mucus sample is taken and examined under a microscope. The clinic is looking to see whether there are any sperm in the mucus, whether they are dead, or whether they are just shaking rather than moving forward. If a man has active, healthy sperm when he gives a sperm sample, and yet in the post-coital test the sperm are dead, then something is obviously happening once the sperm are inside the vagina. The test needs to be performed precisely at the right time of the cycle and it is possible to get a number of false results. This means that it has to be repeated, if it looks as if the woman is killing off her partner's sperm.

There are not many clinics who still do this test and it is interesting that a study published in the *British Medical Journal* in 1998 came to the conclusion that 'Routine use of the post-coital test in infertility investigations leads to more tests and treatments but has no significant effect on the pregnancy rate'.[173] The researchers took couples who were attending an infertility clinic and then split them randomly into two groups. One group had all the usual fertility investigations plus the post-coital test and the other group just the fertility investigations without the post-coital. At the end of the study there was no difference in the number of pregnancies between the two groups, and yet the group having the post-coital test were given more fertility treatments on the basis of their post-coital results.

Sperm Penetration Assay or 'Hamster' Test

This is a test which uses hamster eggs to see whether the sperm can penetrate the eggs. Human sperm are able to penetrate hamster eggs but they cannot (thankfully!) develop into embryos. For the test the zona pellucida (outer layer) of the hamster eggs is removed and the doctors observe how many sperm can penetrate each egg. I doubt the value of this test because if the outer layer of the egg has been removed then it does not replicate the situation between a man and woman, where the sperm has to penetrate the outer layer of the egg for fertilisation to take place. It also suggests that you can compare a woman's egg and a hamster's egg. This test may result in totally worthless information and also involves the unnecessary use of another animal.

White Blood Cells

Immature sperm appear as round cells in the semen before they develop into their characteristic tadpole-like shape. White blood cells are also round and it is not easy to distinguish the two in a sample so special stains are used. It is important to know whether white blood cells are present because they can cause infertility. They could indicate an infection in the urinary tract. If white blood cells are noticed then further investigations are needed to rule out ordinary bacteria or an infection like chlamydia (see Chapter 17).

Hormone Tests

Hormones may be tested and these could include FSH, LH, prolactin, testosterone and thyroid hormones. If FSH levels are high, it may indicate that there is a problem with sperm production in the testes. Giving high doses of testosterone as a medication can actually reduce the sperm count; so we come back once again to the idea of balance, with the hormone needing to be just right, neither too high nor too low. Some medications, such as clomiphene citrate and tamoxifen, have been used to treat male infertility but they are controversial and we do not know how beneficial they are.

Conclusion

If these tests on you or your partner show a definite reason why you are not conceiving (such as blocked fallopian tubes or a low sperm count) you should be referred on for further investigations. Whatever treatment you and your partner have, it will be much more effective if you first put the fertility-boosting recommendations outlined in Section 2 into practice.

CHAPTER 17

Infections Which Can Affect Both Male and Female Fertility

Since the advent of the Pill in the 1960s, sex before marriage has become acceptable. Nowadays serial monogamy (being faithful to one partner before moving onto the next) is often the norm but can mean a number of sexual partners in any person's lifetime. With the use of the Pill (not a barrier method), and the increase in sexual partners, has come a dramatic increase in sexually transmitted diseases. The classical venereal diseases, such as syphilis and gonorrhoea, are in decline – due to early detection and treatment – but their place has been taken by a group of other infectious agents.

A number of these infections can actually stop you getting pregnant and may even cause a miscarriage. They can also drastically affect your partner's sperm.

It is therefore essential that both of you go for an infection screening *before* you try to conceive, especially if there has been a previous miscarriage. Some problems (like toxoplasmosis) are not sexually transmitted but should still be screened for, as they can cause problems once pregnant (see below). A routine screening should also include rubella (German measles) so that you know you are immune before getting pregnant. A number of the infections, as well as affecting your fertility, can pose a serious problem once you are pregnant, and that is why they must be treated before conception.

Infections to be Screened For Before Conception

Chlamydia

This 'infertility time bomb' (discussed in Chapter 3) needs to be checked out for both you and your partner.

Cytomegalovirus (CMV)

CMV, which is caused by a herpes virus, affects a man's fertility by reducing his sperm count.[174]

As well as affecting fertility, it has other far-reaching effects if not picked up before conception. It has been estimated that every year a minimum of 5,000 babies are born in America with some degree of brain damage associated with CMV infection and up to 600 children in the UK. If the baby is infected in the womb, CMV can cause a range of symptoms, including jaundice, eye infections, hearing loss, small for dates, feeding difficulties, and failure to thrive.[175]

The greatest risk to the foetus is when infection occurs during the first 12 weeks of pregnancy. CMV has also been linked to a risk of miscarriage.[176]

CMV is excreted in saliva and urine, so pregnant women and women trying to conceive should avoid kissing and cuddling young children (the incidence is highest in the first few years of life). However if someone has been infected once that provides lifelong immunity.

Mycoplasmas

Mycoplasma hominis and *Ureaplasma urealyticum* are small organisms which are very common in all of us but found in higher quantities in couples who are not conceiving.

In the lab, mycoplasmas (including *Mycoplasma hominis* and *Ureaplasma urealyticum*) have to be grown on a special culture and whether they are tested or not can literally come down to a question of cost. For this reason they are not routinely tested on the NHS and most couples will need to go privately. But, as you will see, it is very important that, as a couple (whether trying to conceive or having experienced a previous miscarriage), you are screened for these very small pathogens.

In some clinics, when a sperm sample is analysed it is also cultured to see whether any ureaplasma is present. This is because the presence of this infection can affect the quality of the sample, in some cases creating adhesions within the sperm. It has been found that the higher the number of ureaplasmas in the semen, the lower the zinc concentration.[177] And we have seen how crucial good levels of zinc are for fertility.

The same study also found that the higher the number of ureaplasmas in the semen, the lower the fructose content. Fructose is a sugar normally found in semen. The absence of fructose in the semen can mean that the seminal vesicles are blocked, stopping both sperm and fructose from getting through. Some researchers have gone so far as to say that ureaplasmas are associated with male infertility,[178] because when men were treated for the infection there was a significant improvement in the motility of their sperm.

The increase in these infections may be due to changes in sexual attitudes and the fact that certain conditions may increase their growth. For instance, it is known that mycoplasma proliferates when the Pill is used.[179]

Unfortunately if a pregnant woman has a ureaplasma infection she can pass it on to her baby. Some interesting research, published in the *New Scientist* magazine in 1997, showed that if babies were infected by *Ureaplasma urealyticum* in the womb then they were more likely to develop asthma in later life. The researchers suggested that asthma could be prevented in some children if the parent were treated before conception.

Rubella (German Measles)

German measles contracted during childhood is a mild disease; and, once infected, the person builds up antibodies which give lifelong immunity to the illness. These antibodies can be measured by a blood test and the woman then knows whether she is 'rubella immune'. The risk of contracting German measles during pregnancy is not to the mother but to the baby. If the mother develops this illness during the first 12 weeks of pregnancy, there is up to five times greater a chance of the baby being born with congenital abnormalities (such as deafness, blindness and heart disease) or being miscarried.

If the woman finds out that she is not rubella immune then she may opt to be immunised before embarking on a pregnancy. One woman I know of, who did not want to be immunised, used a homeopathic remedy to which her body produced the rubella antibodies when subsequently measured on a blood test.

Toxoplasmosis

Toxoplasmosis is an infection of the parasite Toxoplasma gondii which is found in most animals but the only reproductive host is the cat, which acquires the cysts by eating infected birds and mice. It can be transmitted to humans by contact with cat litter, eating raw or partially cooked meat, drinking contaminated water and in unpasteurised dairy products.

If a woman acquires toxoplasmosis during pregnancy, the baby is usually infected in 45 per cent of cases and it is a very serious disease for the foetus. The risk to the baby is greater in the first trimester (first 12 weeks) of pregnancy, when an infection of toxoplasma can cause hydrocephalus (accumulation of fluid on the brain), eye problems, convulsions, blindness and brain damage. Toxoplasmosis can also increase the risk of an early or late miscarriage.

In France pregnant women are routinely tested for toxoplasmosis, sometimes as often as once a month. If a pregnant woman becomes infected then, depending on the stage of pregnancy, advice is given as to the course of action. In this country, the Royal College of Obstetricians and Gynaecologists have concluded that routine screening of toxoplasmosis for pregnant women is not 'appropriate',[180] perhaps due to financial constraints. Once infected with toxoplasmosis, the person acquires life-long immunity.

Prevention is the best approach and that means that, up to four months before pregnancy and during pregnancy, the woman must not handle cat litter. If this is impossible then disposable gloves should be worn. Gloves should also be worn while gardening and hands should be washed thoroughly after changing cat litter, gardening and handling raw meat. If you eat meat only eat it when it is well cooked, wash all fruit and vegetables thoroughly to remove soil, avoid unpasteurised dairy foods such as milk and cheese, and wash your hands before eating.

Genital Herpes

This virus is sexually transmitted. Once acquired, it can come and go, with attacks varying from slight red bumps to blisters. If a woman gets herpes for the first time during the early part of pregnancy it can increase the risk of miscarriage by up to 25 per cent. If herpes is active when the woman gets to term then she is usually offered a Caesarean. This is because, if delivered vaginally, the baby could contract herpes during the delivery and there is a possibility of brain damage, blindness or death.

Gardnerella

This vaginal infection, gardnerella vaginalis, needs to be cleared up before conception. It can cause a burning sensation and also a grey or yellow discharge with a fishy smell.

Group B Haemolytic Streptococci

This is a very common bacteria but it has links with premature rupture of the membranes and premature birth.[181] If this infection is present during birth the mother needs to have antibiotics to prevent the infection spreading to her baby.

General Uterine Infections

Doctors suspect that infections of the uterus could play a crucial role in very early deliveries (before 32 weeks). Uterine infections accelerate the disintegration of the protective membrane in which the baby is encased. Then, a few weeks after the onset of disintegration, the infections cause the uterus to begin contracting. However, as the membranes fall apart, a protein called fibronectin is released. This can be detected using a high vaginal swab (spotting it early would allow doctors to treat the infections using a drug called metronidazole). In a 1998 study, women who were at high risk of pre-term delivery, and were screened for asymptomatic bacteria (an infection causing no symptoms), were given metronidazole and this significantly reduced the incidence of premature birth and also low birthweight.[182]

Of course, in an ideal world, it would be better for women to be screened for this bacteria before conception so that they did not need treatment while pregnant.

Candida

Candida albicans (often called thrush) is a yeast which occurs naturally in the gut, in the skin and in the vagina and is usually controlled by other bacteria. It may not be stopping you conceiving but if you are aiming to optimise your health before conception then it is well worth eliminating it. When the immune system is compromised, say because of illness or bad diet, the proportions of the different bacteria can alter, allowing candida to grow out of control. When antibiotics are given for infection they do not discriminate between the 'good' bacteria in the body and the 'bad' bacteria, they just wipe out everything. In this situation, there are not enough of the 'good' bacteria to keep the candida under control and it can overgrow. Previous use of the Pill can also cause problems with candida,[183] and so can long-term steroid or antibiotic use.

The main symptoms of vaginal thrush are a thick, white, sticky discharge with soreness and irritation. Men can also experience a discharge from the penis with soreness or redness.

Candida is often carried in the digestive system and can give rise to symptoms such as food cravings (especially for sugar and bread), fatigue, bloated stomach with excessive flatulence, feeling spaced out and feeling drunk on a small amount of alcohol. For these symptoms it is best to consult a nutritional therapist (see Useful Addresses).

If you are susceptible to vaginal thrush, prevention is best. Wear cotton underwear and looser-fitting clothes because the yeast grows in a warm, moist environment. Have a break from using tampons and use sanitary towels instead. Avoid perfumed soaps and bubble baths. Use a few drops of tea tree oil in the bath to act as an anti-fungal. Take a good probiotic (the opposite of an antibiotic) which will help to recolonise the gut flora. For example, you could buy a good acidophilus supplement, made by a company such as BioCare or Solgar (see Useful Addresses) and keep it in the fridge.

Infections to be Avoided Once You are Pregnant

Listeria

Listeria is a bacteria that is present in animals and soil. In men and non-pregnant women the infection is mild but in pregnant women it can cause a late miscarriage. To avoid listeria, do not eat soft cheeses such as Brie, Camembert and blue-veined cheeses, meat pâtés, undercooked meat, ready-to-eat poultry (unless thoroughly reheated), soft whipped ice creams that come out of machines, unpasteurised dairy products and ready-prepared salads in sealed bags.

Salmonella

One of the commonest causes of food poisoning, salmonella can cause severe diarrhoea and vomiting. It does not seem to harm the developing baby but a fever accompanying the salmonella may cause a miscarriage. Make sure that all poultry and eggs are thoroughly cooked and avoid eating anything that contains raw eggs (like mayonnaise).

> **TIPS TO AVOID FOOD POISONING**
>
> • Wash hands before preparing food and in between handling raw and cooked food.
> • Keep worktops clean, and wash chopping boards as you go.
> • Wash utensils used for raw foods before they are used on other food.
> • Keep the temperature in your fridge lower than 5°C and the freezer below −18°C.
> • Prepare and store raw and cooked food separately.
> • Keep pets away from food.
> • Do not prepare food for other people if you have any symptoms of food poisoning.
> • Don't overfill the fridge, as this can stop air circulating which could increase the temperature inside.
> • Put leftovers back in the fridge as soon as possible but wait until they cool down.
> • If using leftovers, heat through properly.
> • Thoroughly cook meat and poultry so there are no pink bits.

Infections That Need to be Screened For in Both the Man and the Woman

These include:

- Cytomegalovirus (CMG)
- Mycoplasmas/ureaplasmas
- Chlamydia
- Anaerobic bacteria
- Group B haemolytic streptococci
- Gardnerella vaginalis
- Klebsiella
- Toxoplasmosis
- Candida

The woman also needs to ensure rubella immunity which your GP can organise.

Some GP practices can organise the screening; otherwise many hospitals have a genito-urinary clinic which will test for most of these infections. A number of clinics are extremely helpful if you mention that this is for pre-conception screening. It is not necessary to have a doctor's referral for these clinics and the results are given back to you.

If you have a positive test result for a particular infection, get it treated and then go back for a re-test to make sure it has been eliminated.

SECTION 4

MEDICAL TREATMENT – ASSISTED CONCEPTION

❀

You may have followed the guidelines in Section 2 for several months but still not conceived, or you may have specific medical problems which mean that you require assisted conception. Either way, there is no reason to feel embarrassed or depressed or that you have somehow 'failed'. Thousands of people have fertility treatment each year, and the changes you have already made will make a big difference to your chances of conceiving.

The fact is that couples who have followed the Four-Month Preconception Plan (see Section 6) before having fertility treatment have a significantly higher success rate. A healthy diet and lifestyle puts your body in a much better position to tolerate the drug treatments and medical interventions involved in fertility treatments. It also makes a crucial difference to the future health of your child, for the following reasons.

Our society has the technology to help women and men conceive who otherwise would not have done so. Sometimes a woman is not conceiving for a very good reason. For instance, she may be underweight and undernourished – actually a perfectly natural reason which protects both her and the species. However, drugs are now available that can make her ovulate and conceive, no matter what the state of her underlying health. So it is possible to 'correct' the infertility and then produce a baby of low birthweight, with all the associated health problems (see Chapter 23).

Britain has the most appalling record for low birthweight, the same as poverty-stricken Albania. We now know how much influence birthweight has on the future health of the child. Yet our childhood death rate is worse than in Slovenia. On the other hand, getting a woman into optimum health might have corrected the fertility problem without the use of any drugs and resulted in a proper weight healthy baby. Of course, there are lots of cases where fertility treatment is appropriate – if you have blocked fallopian tubes for instance, or if your partner has had undescended testes when younger. These cases are different but both partners should still get themselves into optimum health before trying to conceive.

Side-effects

Fertility treatments can involve taking large quantities of powerful drugs, many of which may have side-effects. And studies have shown that the negative effect of a drug can be enhanced if there are nutrient deficiencies.

The classic example is thalidomide, the infamous drug given to pregnant women in the 1960s for their morning sickness, which resulted in thousands of birth defects. When tested on well-fed rats, thalidomide had no negative effects at all. Even a substantial dose of thalidomide did not result in malformations in the offspring. But as soon as the rats were made deficient in a number of vitamins and given the thalidomide, many of the offspring miscarried or were born congenitally malformed.[184]

The same happened with zinc. When there was a zinc deficiency the thalidomide immediately became teratogenic (literally 'monster forming') but it wasn't when zinc was plentiful.[185] So if you know you are going to have drug treatment you should try to lessen the possibility of side-effects by ensuring that you are properly nourished. Of course there is another concern. If drugs are only tested routinely on well-fed animals do we really get to see the possible side-effects of a particular drug on less well-nourished humans?

CHAPTER 18

Where Can You Get Help?

It is not easy to get fertility treatment on the NHS and sometimes only drug treatments are available. A study carried out by University College Hospital and Medical School in London showed that 75 per cent of couples end up on long NHS waiting lists and would choose to go privately if medical insurance companies would foot the bill. The best system is in France where the state pays for four IVF cycles. In Germany the couple are allowed four and 30 per cent of the cost is paid for by the state and the rest made up by the insurance companies. The availability of NHS treatment can often depend on where you live. There are no central guidelines. Some couples I see have had a number of IUIs (see page 163) on the NHS, and others who have gone privately for IVF have had their fertility drugs funded by their GP. There are also some non-profit-making clinics where the cost is much lower than private IVF clinics.

Choosing a Clinic

In the UK, all clinics offering assisted conception have to be licensed by the HFEA, Human Fertilisation and Embryology Authority (see Useful Addresses). The HFEA produces 'league tables' showing how successful the clinics are – essential reading for all couples deciding where to go for treatment. CHILD (see Useful Addresses) also produces a helpful booklet called *Choosing a Clinic*.

If you are going privately, remember that you are a paying customer and you want the service that suits you best. Some couples prefer a small intimate clinic, where they see the same professionals at each visit. Others prefer a large clinic, headed by a well-known name who you may or may not see. This can be more impersonal and it is likely that you will see different doctors each time you go. Some couples say that, in a big clinic, they feel as if they are on a conveyor belt. Others prefer this. It's best to get brochures from a number of clinics and visit up to three of them to decide whether you would feel comfortable being treated there. Convenience also has to be a factor because you will be going quite a few times and you don't want to travel too far.

Success Rates

Each clinic releases its own statistics but you can't really compare them because they are often calculated differently so that you're not comparing 'like with like'. The HFEA guide, on the other hand, presents standardised statistics, the most important of which is the 'take-home baby rate' per treatment cycle. If the pregnancy rates alone are compared these can look very impressive. But these would tell you nothing about what happened later – the rates of miscarriage, ectopic (tubal) pregnancies, and any other problems that meant the pregnancy did not continue.

The other point to bear in mind is that, since the publication of these HFEA 'league tables', some clinics have become more selective in their patients. If they take everybody, including 'older' women and other complicated cases, their position in the league tables may be affected.

Some clinics are more honest and upfront than others in telling a couple that, in view of their medical history, they have an extremely small chance of getting pregnant. Others will take anybody who is willing to pay.

Useful Questions to Ask the Clinic

- What tests and treatments are provided?
- Do they specialise in any particular type of infertility?
- Is there a waiting list?
- Are there any restrictions (e.g. due to age or previous treatments)?
- How often will you have to attend the clinic?
- Is counselling provided and is it included in the treatment costs?
- Are there any hidden costs, such as diagnostic tests or anaesthetic charges?
- What is the up-to-date take-home baby rate?
- What is their success rate like for a woman the same age as you? (Some clinics have more experience with 'older' women.)

Ask each clinic the same questions and compare the answers. You can visit them or some clinics will answer these questions over the phone. The HFEA publishes a patient's handbook which will help you to compare the different clinics. You really want to get as much information as possible so that you can get the best treatment to suit your individual needs.

Before You Start

Embarking on IVF treatment is a big step, both financially and emotionally, so it needs to be thought out carefully. Many couples are not aware of the amount of time it is going to take up, the physical effects of the drugs on the woman's body, and the emotional roller-coaster that it will put them through.

The full financial cost may not be clear at the outset. One couple I know recently had a cycle of IVF treatment that cost them £6,000 instead of the more usual £2,000–£3,000 because so many drugs were required in order to get an effect. So beware of extra costs that may only become apparent once the cycle begins.

The success rate for IVF is around 20 per cent, which means that 80 per cent of treatment cycles will fail. This success rate is the same for each cycle and is not dependent on how many cycles you have had already. The odds are the same as if you toss a coin. If you have tossed four heads, there is still a 50:50 chance that the next one is going to be another head.

Some couples can feel under pressure to have one IVF cycle after another. Sometimes this pressure comes from the clinics, especially if the woman is 'older'. However, with the quantities of drugs that are used and the emotional ups and downs that can be experienced, together with the effects of these drugs on your system, it is better to have a break, say two or three months, between attempts and let your body get back to a natural cycle before it is bombarded again.

CHAPTER 19

What are the Different Types of Fertility Treatment?

Drugs for Inducing Ovulation

This is usually the first line of treatment if it is discovered that you are not ovulating but your fallopian tubes and your partner's sperm are normal. A number of drug treatments are available, designed to stimulate ovulation, correct the hormone balance and ensure the release of an egg. These drugs do not actually make you more fertile: they only work during the month they are being taken.

Clomiphene Citrate

Clomiphene citrate stimulates ovulation if you are not ovulating and it is also used if you have infrequent periods and long cycles. It is taken for five days early on in the cycle.

This drug should not be used for more than six cycles, as there is an increased risk of ovarian cancer with 12 or more cycles of clomiphene treatment.[186]

One of the side-effects of clomiphene can be multiple births. Although this drug is easy to administer, since it is taken by mouth and could be given by a GP, the Royal College of Obstetricians and Gynaecologists recommends that it should only be given where ultrasound monitoring can be done at the same time. Monitoring also means that the dose can be altered, depending on your response to the drug. You may suffer other side-effects from clomiphene, such as bowel upsets, bloating, headache, dizziness, breast discomfort, blurred vision, hot flushes and depression. Unfortunately clomiphene also increases the miscarriage rate.

Human Chorionic Gonadotrophin (hCG)

This hormone should be produced naturally in the early stages of pregnancy. It works in the same way as luteinising hormone (LH) by causing the dominant follicle to release its egg. It can be used in conjunction with clomiphene. This is given as an injection and there are no known side-effects.

Human Menopausal Gonadotrophin (hMG)

This is one of the most potent ovulation drugs in use, and is derived from the urine of post-menopausal women. It combines both FSH and LH and is given by injection. This drug is often used for women who have not had any success with clomiphene. It is also used for women who have amenorrhoea (no periods). There is an increased risk of multiple births so careful monitoring is needed.

As with clomiphene, there can be a higher miscarriage risk and also premature labour. Mood swings, depression and breast tenderness may also be experienced. There are dangers of hyperstimulation, where the ovaries can become enlarged and cause abdominal pain. Extreme hyperstimulation can be life-threatening and fluid accumulates in the chest and abdominal cavity. You should be monitored closely, and doctors will withhold treatment if there are too many follicles present or if your oestrogen level is too high. In this case, the cycle will be abandoned.

Follicle Stimulating Hormone (FSH)

Like hMG, this drug is also derived from the urine of post-menopausal women (often nuns for ease of collection), and is given as an injection. Because the demand for it has been so high, there is also a genetically engineered form of FSH called recombinant human FSH. This medication does not really contain any LH and it can only be used by women who have adequate amounts of their own LH. It can be useful for women with polycystic ovarian syndrome (PCOS) because they tend to have high LH levels. It is possible to have a kit with this drug so that you can self-inject under the skin.

Bromocriptine

This drug is used if a woman secretes too much prolactin from the pituitary gland. Prolactin is the same hormone that stimulates breast milk and can stop ovulation and periods because it inhibits the release of FSH and LH. Excess prolactin can also be caused by a benign tumour within the pituitary gland so cases of high prolactin should be investigated fully. This drug is given in tablet form and can cause nausea, headache, dizziness, fainting and decreased blood pressure. Carbergoline is a newer drug for treating high levels of prolactin and it has fewer side-effects than bromocriptine.

Gonadotropin Releasing Hormone (GnRH)

GnRH is released naturally from the hypothalamus in the brain in small amounts every 90 minutes. This pulsing effect releases both FSH and LH from the pituitary gland. If the patient has a deficiency of GnRH then FSH and LH will not be secreted. When women lose large amounts of weight quickly (or if they have anorexia) the secretion of GnRH decreases, stopping ovulation and causing infertility. Because GnRH works in a pulsing rhythm, it has to be given in the same way to mimic the natural cycle. This means that the woman has to wear an automatic pump 24 hours a day; at intervals of 90 minutes the pump releases the GnRH which goes to a needle inserted under the skin. Side-effects can include headaches and nausea. And there is a slight risk of multiple pregnancy.

Gonadotropin Releasing Hormone (GnRH) Analogues

These are synthetic hormones that work in a very different way to GnRH. They can be given as an injection or as a nasal spray. Because it gives a constant dose of synthetic GnRH to the hypothalamus, instead of the pulsed GnRH (above), the pituitary stops releasing both FSH and LH. This in turn stops the production of hormones by the ovaries, so oestrogen levels drop. These analogues are often used in IVF treatments because they are believed to result in more mature eggs (by stopping the release of LH which could cause the follicles to release eggs before they were ready). Side-effects include headaches, mood swings, vaginal dryness and insomnia. These analogues are often used to treat endometriosis and fibroids.

Drugs for Male Infertility

There are also a number of drug treatments your partner can be offered if problems are found with the quantity or quality of his semen.

hCG and hMG

These two drugs (the same ones as those mentioned above) can be used either separately or together for men who are deficient in LH and FSH, which in turn causes problems with sperm production. Men with a lack of GnRH can benefit from this treatment or the use of pulsing GnRH. It is interesting that many of these men (and women with a lack of GnRH) may have lost their sense of smell, which can also indicate a deficiency of zinc, a vital nutrient for fertility (see page 82).

Bromocriptine

Men can also have high levels of prolactin which can cause loss of libido and impotence. This drug lowers prolactin, just as it does in women.

Clomiphene or tamoxifen

These are both anti-oestrogens which have been given to men where no hormone imbalances have been found but the sperm count is low. However, these drugs do *not* have product licences for male infertility. And the Royal College of Obstetricians and Gynaecologists states that the use of these drugs has been shown to be ineffective in treating male infertility.[187]

Testosterone

This is another hormone which is of questionable value in fertility treatment. It is often given where there is no hormone imbalance but there is a problem with the sperm count. Proper development of sperm is dependent on high levels of testosterone and the amount that would need to be taken orally to get the required effect could have a destructive effect on the liver. Also, giving testosterone creates a vicious circle by decreasing levels of FSH and LH, causing further problems with sperm production. The Royal College of Obstetricians and Gynaecologists, reviewing the papers on the use of testosterone, felt that there was no evidence for effectiveness and even if it had a placebo effect the dangers of using it were too great.[188]

Corticosteroids

These are sometimes used for men who have anti-sperm antibodies. But there is no real evidence for the effectiveness of this treatment.[189] The side-effects can include weight gain, dyspepsia, facial flushing, bloating, skin rashes, irritability and insomnia.

Case History

Jennifer was 34 and had been trying to conceive for the ten years since she had been married, but her husband had been told that he had a low sperm count. Two varicoceles (see page 21) were diagnosed and operated on but this did not improve his sperm count. Four years previously he had been diagnosed with testicular cancer and one testicle had been removed, followed by radiotherapy and chemotherapy. Some sperm had been frozen before treatment. Jennifer had tried two ICSI treatments (see page 168) but they had been unsuccessful. She contacted me in August 1997 on her own, as the couple lived abroad and she was going back straight away. Her nutritional analysis showed very low levels of magnesium and high levels of copper (common after fertility treatment). I gave her a programme of supplements and suggested changes in her diet which she followed for the four months of the Preconception Plan (see Section 6). At the end of December the same year I received a fax from her telling me she was five weeks pregnant. She now has a lovely baby girl.

Assisted Conception Techniques

Looked at simply, these procedures can firstly increase the number of eggs released in any one cycle. (In IUI it can be two to three eggs. In IVF it can be two to eight eggs.) Secondly, these techniques can shorten the distance between your eggs and your partner's sperm.

Fertilisation can take place inside or outside the body, depending on which procedure is used:

- In IUI the sperm are put in the womb so fertilisation is inside.
- In GIFT the sperm and egg are mixed together outside the body but fertilisation takes place inside.
- In IVF the sperm and egg are put next to each other in the dish so fertilisation is outside.
- In ICSI the sperm is put inside the egg so fertilisation is outside.

There are a number of different assisted conception treatments available. I will start with the 'low tech' ones and go on to the more complicated treatments. Unless there is a medical reason not to, I suggest you embark on assisted conception by trying the low tech treatments first. The others are really a last resort. But your choice may be determined by your medical history. For instance, if you have blocked tubes you will need to go straight to IVF, while a partner with an extremely low sperm count will need to go straight to ICSI. Age is another factor. After the age of 35 the success rates for all procedures decline. As IUI has a lower success rate than IVF, a woman over 35 will probably be better advised to go straight for IVF.

Intra-uterine Insemination (IUI)

IUI is a procedure that puts your partner's sperm directly into your womb at a much higher level than can be achieved during intercourse, to improve the chances of fertilisation.

Who Should Have It?

If you have been given a diagnosis of unexplained infertility, you are under the age of 35, and there seems to be no medical or physical reason why you and your partner are not conceiving, IUI should be the first assisted conception treatment offered.

IUI can be used if you have a problem with ovulation because stimulatory drugs can be given at the same time. Stimulatory drugs are often used anyway to encourage two or three eggs to mature and to increase the chance of the technique working.

IUI can also be used if the man produces an anti-sperm antibody which usually means that his sperm will not penetrate the cervical mucus of the woman.

Again, IUI can be used if a post-coital test has shown that your mucus is hostile to your partner's sperm (see page 142).

IUI can be used with donor sperm if your partner is infertile or has a hereditary disease. However, donor insemination is an emotional issue – particularly for your partner who may feel he has 'failed' as a man. There may also be religious concerns and you should be counselled if donor insemination is required to enable you to conceive. Using a friend or family member as a donor is not usually advised because of the possibility of future problems as the child grows up.

What Happens?

The aim is to get your partner's sperm high into your womb at ovulation when you are most fertile.

You will both have to go to the clinic and your partner will be asked to produce a fresh semen sample. His semen may be 'washed' in a special fluid and centrifuged so that the weaker sperm are filtered out. Alternatively a 'swim up' test can filter out weaker sperm. Sometimes a 'split ejaculate' is used because the first part of the ejaculate contains many more sperm.

Ultrasound is used to track the development of the follicles so that the sperm can be inserted at precisely the right time. This tracking is also important so that, if there is overstimulation from any of the drugs and the possibility of a multiple birth, the procedure can be abandoned.

IUI may be a bit embarrassing but it is not at all painful. No anaesthetic is needed and the sperm is placed high in the womb through a fine catheter. You will have to rest for a little while afterwards.

Success Rate

When there are no medical reasons for infertility IUI has a good success rate – around 15 per cent before the age of 35.

If you have been given a diagnosis of unexplained infertility, and you know your tubes are clear and that your partner's sperm is healthy, IUI may be the first assisted conception treatment you are offered.

I feel that it is not offered enough, however, and that too many couples with unexplained infertility go straight to IVF treatment without trying IUI or other options first. Maybe I am being cynical but IVF is more lucrative for the clinics than IUI, which costs only one-tenth of the amount.

In-vitro Fertilisation (IVF)

IVF is a technique for fertilising your eggs with your partner's sperm outside your body – hence the use of the phrase 'test tube babies'. The fertilised egg is then implanted back into your womb.

Who Should Have It?

IVF may be used as a last resort by couples who have had unexplained fertility for a number of years. It is often chosen if the woman has damaged fallopian tubes or other specific problems which mean that normal fertilisation cannot take place.

IVF is also an option if there are any other problems and you are over the age of 35.

What Happens?

In order to prepare you and your body for this procedure, GnRH analogues are given, either as a nasal spray or daily injection, in order to work as an anti-hormone to put you into a temporary menopausal state. This is called down-regulation and stops your own hormones interfering with the IVF treatment. Another fertility drug, FSH or hMG, is then given in the form of injections to stimulate several follicles to develop.

Once there are enough follicles of the correct size (as monitored by ultrasound), you are given an injection of hCG which primes the eggs before they are collected.

Around 34–38 hours later the eggs are collected through the vagina, using an aspiration needle guided by ultrasound. You may be sedated for this procedure or have a general anaesthetic.

Your partner provides a fresh semen sample, which is treated as in IUI (above), and up to 100,000 sperm are mixed with each egg. The aim is to collect about 20 eggs. The ones that are fertilised, and start to divide well, will be chosen to go back inside the womb. This takes place two or three days later and the embryos are transferred into the womb via the cervix, using a soft catheter.

Only a maximum of three embryos can be implanted back, according to UK law, and it is hoped that they will implant in the womb. Because the embryos are put directly into the womb, they end up there three or four days earlier than they would do normally. It takes an embryo (fertilised egg) approximately seven days to travel down the fallopian tube before it ends up in the womb.

In order to increase the chances of implantation, the hormone progesterone is given either as pessaries or injections.

Success Rate

Despite all the hype, the IVF success rate is relatively low – only 15–20 per cent.

IVF treatment most commonly fails at the implantation stage. Many couples tell me that everything went really well until they reached this point.

Sometimes the IVF cycle is abandoned because the drugs either failed to stimulate egg production or, at the other extreme, caused hyperstimulation which is potentially dangerous. Sometimes no eggs can be retrieved from the follicles or the quality of the eggs is poor and fertilisation with the sperm is unsuccessful.

Assisted Hatching

In normal pregnancy, a hole is made naturally in the casing of the embryo and the embryo hatches and attaches itself to the lining of the womb. The enzymes present in the fallopian tube that usually soften the casing are not present in IVF because in IVF the embryos are put back straight into the womb. So, if there have been a number of failed attempts at IVF, a technique called assisted hatching may be used, whereby a needle or chemical is used to make a tiny hole in the casing of the embryo.

Frozen Embryos

Extra embryos resulting from the IVF treatment can be frozen if their quality is good. However, under the HFEA Act of 1990, these embryos can only be kept in storage for five years. They do not thaw out well and many have to be discarded. The embryos are stored in liquid nitrogen and, in order to prevent what is called 'cooling injury', as the embryos are thawed out, cryoprotectant chemicals are used. Of course, there are also moral and ethical issues which have to be considered when deciding to freeze embryos, because it is not eggs that are being frozen but a potential baby.

Gamete Intra Fallopian Transfer (GIFT)

Your egg is mixed together (not fertilised) with your partner's sperm and put back into the fallopian tubes so that fertilisation takes place where it would happen naturally anyway.

Who Should Have It?

GIFT can only be used when a woman has open and healthy fallopian tubes.

What Happens?

The use of the drugs is identical to IVF but the difference is that the egg retrieval is done by a laparoscope (telescope) through the abdomen and so a general anaesthetic is needed. A maximum of three eggs are put back in the fallopian tube.

The other difference between GIFT and IVF is that fertilisation, if successful, takes place inside the body. GIFT is more invasive and expensive than IVF.

Success Rate

There are no official success rates for GIFT treatment because it does not come under the HFEA which only monitors techniques involving an embryo outside the body.

One clinic estimates that GIFT is approximately one and a half times more successful than IVF because fertilisation takes place inside your fallopian tubes and the embryo does not reach the womb until approximately seven days later, as nature intended. (As we have seen, IVF fails most commonly at this crucial implantation stage.)

Frozen Eggs

Any excess eggs from a GIFT procedure can be fertilised with the sperm outside the body, as in IVF. This makes it possible to see whether fertilisation actually takes place, and the embryos can be frozen.

GIFT-ET

This is a fairly new technique which is only done by a few clinics but it is well worth asking about because the take-home baby rate can be as high as 41 per cent.

The treatment involves a combination of GIFT and IVF – both procedures are performed in the same cycle. One or two of the eggs collected are mixed with sperm and put back in the fallopian tube, and at the same time one fertilised egg is put back in the womb. This combined technique is proving to be more successful than either one of the treatments on their own. As with GIFT, the woman must have healthy fallopian tubes for this technique to be considered.

Intracytoplasmic Sperm Injection (ICSI)

This involves a single sperm being injected directly into the egg to fertilise it. The embryo is then implanted in the womb.

ICSI developed out of a technique called SUZI (Sub-zonal insemination), where five to ten sperm were injected just underneath the layer of cells, the zona pellucida, that surrounds the egg.

Who Should Have It?

ICSI can be used if your partner's sperm count is so low that IVF is not possible, if he cannot ejaculate, or if he has an obstruction stopping his sperm being released.

What Happens?

You will have to undergo the same preparations with drug treatment and procedures as for IVF (see above).

The human egg is invisible to the naked eye and sperm are minute in comparison to an egg, so ICSI is a very delicate procedure.

For men who can't ejaculate or whose sperm are obstructed, the sperm samples can be drawn off directly from the testes or epididymis. If this does not work then a biopsy is performed, in which fingernail-size pieces are taken from the testes through a tiny incision. The sperm retrieved in this way are not fully developed and may not move.

Success Rate

The success rate for ICSI, 20–25 per cent, is slightly higher than for IVF. This is probably due to the fact that the sperm is injected directly into the egg so the technique is not dependent on how well fertilisation takes place.

Risks

In IVF a number of sperm are put in with the egg, which seems to be able to favour healthy sperm over those that may be defective. In ICSI the egg has no 'choice' because only one sperm is used and inserted directly. Because of this, and the fact that often immature sperm or even sperm cells are used, there have been concerns that ICSI could result in babies being born with chromosome defects or having genetic problems later in life.[190]

Researchers have found that babies born after ICSI are twice as likely to have a major birth defect and 50 per cent more likely to have a minor defect.[191]

It has been suggested that men go for karyotyping (chromosome evaluation) before they embark on ICSI so that any genetic causes of their infertility can be ruled out. If there is a genetic cause for the man's infertility, the man and his partner should be counselled as to whether it is right for ICSI to proceed because of the possibility of passing on problems to the baby. Boys born following ICSI might, for instance, be infertile and need ICSI themselves in order to conceive.

It is important to know why the man is infertile, especially if he is producing no sperm. If there are chromosome problems in the man then it is also likely that the miscarriage rate could be high after ICSI.

Sometimes we can't conceive because nature has a fail-safe mechanism to protect the survival of the fittest. Even though we now have the technology to override this, there are some situations where the consequences for the baby should be thought through carefully.

Reasons to be Cautious About Fertility Treatment

We are going against nature with assisted conception techniques like IVF because the body is being asked to mature a great number of eggs in one cycle. (Normally only two at the most would ever be released at the same time.)

The question which is often asked, and rightly so, is: what are the long-term effects of taking these drugs on you and the baby that is conceived? And what are the effects if you have 12 attempts at IVF in an effort to conceive a child?

These questions are not easy to answer at the moment because the first baby born from IVF is only 21. In fact no drugs were used at all to achieve that first success. It was just done with the woman's natural cycle, taking the one egg that was produced. The doctors had used drugs before with their other unsuccessful IVF patients but felt that this was hindering the success of the treatment.

At the moment it is not easy to say what the long-term effect on the 'test tube babies' will be, because they are still growing up. We do not yet know what effects the drugs will have on their fertility, for example.

It stands to reason that bombarding the ovaries with drugs like clomiphene is likely to have a long-term effect on the mother, however. The ovaries are being stimulated in a totally unnatural way and concerns have been expressed about the risk of ovarian cancer. At least one high-profile victim, the late fashion editor Liz Tilberis, believed that her disease was linked in some way to fertility treatments she had had years before.

Ovarian cancer is called the 'silent disease' because it is not usually detected until it is well advanced. There are two theories as to the natural cause of ovarian cancer. One is that each time a woman ovulates there is damage to the surface of the ovary which eventually triggers cancer.[192] This is backed up by research which shows that women who ovulate less, such as those who have quite a few pregnancies and also breastfeed, have a lower rate of ovarian cancer. The other theory is that ovarian cancer is triggered by exposure to gonadotrophin hormones which are also used in IVF treatment.[193]

The scientific results are not conclusive and more long-term research needs to be done. Some studies show that there is an increased risk of ovarian cancer for women who have undergone fertility treatment.[194] Others show no risk.[195]

Conclusion

In the light of all this I think that it is wise to be cautious about any fertility treatments you are offered. They should be regarded as a last resort, once you have really tried the alternatives outlined in this book.

Fertility treatments may involve heavy doses of drugs as well as invasive medical procedures. They can be embarrassing and uncomfortable, and can certainly put a strain on your relationship with your partner. They are by no means an easy option, and that is something to think about and weigh up if you are concerned that following my Four-Month Preconception Plan is too demanding.

If you are in your twenties or early thirties you have enough time to complete the Four-Month Plan and wait a few months for the improvements in your health and fertility to become established. What have you got to lose?

If you are older you should start having tests earlier but, by following the Four-Month Plan, you will be in much better shape whatever choices you finally make.

SECTION 5

WHEN THINGS
GO WRONG

❊

Suffering a miscarriage is one of the most devastating things that can happen to a woman – and to her partner. You may have conceived easily and quickly, with none of the problems we have been discussing in the previous sections, and then had the shock of losing the baby. (Most miscarriages happen in the early weeks.)

Not only have you and your partner suffered a loss but you will obviously be worried about why it happened. You may be concerned that it was somehow your fault or feel that the doctors have made light of a very personal and traumatic event. Above all, you will want to know how you can prevent a miscarriage happening again.

The reason why the medical profession often seems lacking in sympathy is that miscarriages are actually very common. In many cases a woman does not realise that she has had one because it happened before she knew she was pregnant and she might have just thought she had a rather heavy period.

It is estimated that at least a quarter of all pregnancies end in miscarriage, usually before the twelfth week of pregnancy, and often (unknown to the woman) much much earlier. Scientists believe that in many cases these early miscarriages are nature's way of dealing with an abnormal foetus that could not succeed in becoming a healthy baby.

That does not make it any easier to get over a miscarriage. But it does mean that you must not automatically assume that there is something wrong with you or your capacity to sustain a pregnancy. This kind of anxiety causes the kind of stress that can upset your system so much it stops you conceiving again.

What you must do is be positive. Look at all aspects of your health and lifestyle (as described in Section 2) and follow the Four-Month Preconception Plan (Section 6) to give you and your partner the best chance of a successful pregnancy. If you have suffered a miscarriage the doctor will have given you advice on how long you should wait before you try to conceive again.

Use that time to get yourself and your partner really healthy in the way I have outlined. If you do this you will dramatically improve your chances of avoiding another miscarriage when you conceive.

CHAPTER 20

Preventing Miscarriages

What is a Miscarriage?

The medical term for miscarriage is 'spontaneous abortion' and it occurs before week 24 of pregnancy. After 24 weeks, the delivery of a baby which has died is called a stillbirth. Many women do not like the term 'spontaneous abortion' as it reminds them of 'induced abortion' which is the deliberate ending of a pregnancy.

The miscarriage may be complete or incomplete. If it is complete, then the miscarriage has finished and all 'the products of conception' have come away. These include the foetus, placenta and amniotic sac. In an incomplete miscarriage some of these 'products' are left behind and bleeding can continue. In this situation there is always a possible risk of infection if the products are left for any length of time and the woman will be advised to have an ERCP (evacuation of the retained products of conception).

Many women will not notice anything amiss until they have a scan and are then told that the foetus seems to have stopped developing and has died – this is called a 'missed abortion'. They are usually offered a D and C (dilation and curettage) which is a scraping of the womb lining.

In some cases, the fertilised egg (ovum) will not have developed or developed poorly. On a scan, there will be a pregnancy sac but no embryo because the foetus stopped growing very early in pregnancy. The medical term for this is 'blighted ovum'.

What Causes a Miscarriage?

This is still largely an unanswered question. There are medical reasons why some women miscarry and tests can show if these are the reasons. Other women will miscarry and yet all the test results are normal. It is easier for a woman to deal with a miscarriage if there is a reason for it happening, and for something to be done about it so that it doesn't happen again.

Some experts believe that a miscarriage is the most sensitive of all indicators that a woman or her partner have been exposed to an environmental hazard.[196] Others would disagree.

There is certainly a greater risk of miscarriage before week 12 of pregnancy. This is because, until the twelfth week, the embryo is floating unattached in the womb. At the twelfth week, the embryo becomes attached to the placenta instead and the pregnancy is much more firmly established. If a problem occurs after this point, the reasons are usually quite different from those of a miscarriage before the twelfth week.

We know that about one in four pregnancies end in early miscarriages, but should we accept this high rate as 'normal'? Arthritis is very common in our society as we get older; in other cultures it is not. Does this make it 'normal'? Or are there ways of preventing arthritis by looking at our lifestyle?

In the same way, we need to look at all the possible causes of miscarriage (lifestyle factors as well as medical problems) in order to prevent it recurring.

The risk of miscarriage increases as we get older. Before the age of 40 the risk of miscarriage is about 15 per cent and it can rise to around 40 per cent in women over the age of 40, mostly because of genetic abnormalities.

Fibroids

A further complication that comes with age is fibroids. These are non-cancerous growths that grow in or on the wall of the womb and are more common as we get older. They are thought to be oestrogen-dependent, as they can shrink at the menopause. Fibroids are given different names depending on where they grow (see Chapter 15). Fibroids that protrude into the womb (submucosal fibroids) can give the greatest risk of a miscarriage because they may make it difficult for the implanted embryo to develop properly.

Chromosomal Abnormality

This is the most common reason for a miscarriage and is usually the result of a one-off genetic abnormality in the baby that is unlikely to recur. In other words nature is working according to the law of survival of the fittest. When the baby is abnormal it will try to stop that pregnancy continuing.

You and your partner each contribute 23 chromosomes to the baby, making 23 pairs in total. Each chromosome pair determines specific characteristics of your child and geneticists have given a number to each pair. For example, number 23 is the pair which determines the sex of the baby.

Only a small portion of chromosomal abnormalities are inherited and these can be screened. The others can occur before, during and after fertilisation, as the chromosomes divide. It is thought that up to 50 per cent of miscarriages can be due to a genetic abnormality.

The most common chromosomal abnormality diagnosed is where there are three chromosomes in the pair instead of two. Depending on which pair this happens to, it will give rise to a specific abnormality. Not all abnormalities always end in a miscarriage. For instance, Down's Syndrome is caused by an extra chromosome on pair number 21 and for that reason is also called trisomy 21. It is thought that most trisomies are caused by an abnormal division in the egg which occurs before fertilisation.

This may explain why older women have always been thought to have a higher risk of having a Down's Syndrome baby, since older women's eggs are more likely to be abnormal. But the Down's Syndrome Association claims that eight out of ten babies with Down's Syndrome are born to mothers under the age of 35. The extra chromosome can also come from the man's sperm. So, at the moment, scientists do not know for sure what causes Down's Syndrome.

However, there are links between Down's Syndrome and mineral deficiencies. For example, people with Down's Syndrome children have lower levels of zinc and selenium compared with others of the same age.[197] It has also been found that in Down's Syndrome blood levels of the 'antioxidant defence system' enzymes (superoxide dismutase and glutathione peroxidase) are over-produced. Both these enzymes are produced by the body to disarm free radicals. The building blocks for these enzymes include the minerals zinc and selenium.

Selenium is known to protect against chromosome (DNA) damage by protecting the body against toxins and pollutants, and future research may demonstrate the importance of prospective parents having good levels of this mineral in the months before conception when both sperm and eggs are maturing.

The idea that toxin damage could be implicated in Down's has been borne out by a study in the wake of the Chernobyl nuclear disaster. Babies born nine months later showed a six-fold increase in cases of Down's Syndrome.[198] Studies on animals have also shown it is possible to damage the chromosomes by introducing a toxin.[199]

So the opposite may also be true: that you can protect your chromosomes from damage by stopping your intake of all the toxins we have been talking about and making sure that you have enough antioxidants to fight unavoidable pollution (like traffic fumes).

Turner's Syndrome

If one chromosome of the pair is missing the condition is called monosomy. The most common abnormality of this type is where one X (female chromosome) is missing from the sex pair (number 23). This condition is called Turner's syndrome. It does not usually cause a miscarriage but the baby, which is always a girl, will have certain physical characteristics. She can have heart defects and fertility problems, because her ovaries may be absent or fail to develop and because of this she will have under-developed breasts. As she gets older, she will need hormone treatment and counselling.

Inherited Genetic Problems

This is a much less common reason for a miscarriage, and chromosome testing (karyotype analysis) would be recommended for both partners where couples have experienced recurrent miscarriages. One of the most common structural changes in chromosomes is translocation, where part of one chromosome comes away and reattaches to a different chromosome.

Some gene defects can cause miscarriages but it is more likely that the genetic problem will cause abnormalities in the baby, such as cystic fibrosis or muscular dystrophy.

Other Causes

Infections

This could be a one-off situation where the mother has caught a severe infection during the early part of pregnancy and it is unlikely to recur in a subsequent pregnancy. Or the miscarriage could be due to a genito-urinary infection which needs to be treated before conceiving again to prevent another miscarriage. Mr Ronnie Lamont, consultant obstetrician and gynaecologist at Northwick Park Hospital, believes that bacterial vaginosis may trigger miscarriage or premature birth. A study he conducted with 800 women found that those with bacterial vaginosis had five times the risk of late miscarriage (16–24 weeks), and those who delivered early (24–37 weeks) also had the infection. Other infections that can cause a miscarriage are discussed in Section 3.

Some infections do not cause a miscarriage but a congenital abnormality (where the baby is born with a defect or malformation). For example, German measles (rubella), contracted in early pregnancy, can lead to babies born with congenital blindness, deafness and mental retardation. A simple blood test can tell you whether you are rubella immune, meaning that you have had German measles or have been vaccinated in the past and so have rubella antibodies in your blood to prevent you from getting it again.

Fertility Drugs

One of the most commonly prescribed medicines for fertility problems is clomiphene citrate which is used to induce ovulation. Ironically, though it may increase a woman's chances of conceiving, it also increases the chance of a miscarriage by 20–30 per cent.[200] It is thought that the clomiphene can interfere with the womb lining, preventing the fertilised egg from implanting. Other techniques used to induce ovulation, like gonadotrophin treatment, can also increase the miscarriage rate.

Weight Problems

It is important not to be underweight or overweight when trying to conceive. Girls don't begin to menstruate until their bodies are composed of at least 17 per cent fat. Studies have shown that 50 per cent of women who have a Body Mass Index (BMI) below 20.7 are infertile.[201] A BMI of approximately 23–24 would be ideal for conception. (To calculate your BMI, see page 58)

Women with anorexia and girls who exercise to the extreme (such as athletes and gymnasts) can lose their menstrual cycle because of the reduction of fat and therefore become technically infertile temporarily.

At the other extreme, it is known that obesity increases the risk of miscarriage.[202]

Problems with excess weight can also be linked with polycystic ovaries

(PCO) which can make conception more difficult (see Chapter 15). Miscarriages are more likely to occur in women with this condition. However, in a study of women with PCO who were asked to change their diet, the rate of miscarriages dropped from 75 per cent to 18 per cent for the same women once they had lost weight.[203]

Hormonal Problems

Luteinising hormone (LH) controls the development and release of the egg from the ovary. Women who have high levels of this hormone in the first half of their menstrual cycle seem to have a greater risk of miscarriage. In addition, women with polycystic ovary syndrome (PCOS) have raised levels of LH.

Progesterone is the hormone which maintains the pregnancy during the first few weeks. After the egg has been released from the ovary, the ruptured follicle then develops into the corpus luteum which produces progesterone. If the egg is not fertilised, after 14 days the corpus luteum withers, progesterone levels fall and a period occurs. If the egg is fertilised and the embryo implants successfully and starts to produce another hormone hCG (human chorionic gonadotrophin) then the corpus luteum gets the message to continue producing progesterone. Without sufficient levels of progesterone, the pregnancy cannot continue, and that is why anti-progesterone drugs are now used to terminate an early pregnancy without the need for an operation.

Because of this obvious link between progesterone and maintaining pregnancy, many doctors give progesterone as injections or pessaries to prevent a miscarriage. But Professor Lesley Regan, in her excellent book *Miscarriage*, states that 'Injections of hormone, in the early weeks of a pregnancy at risk, may prolong the miscarriage but they cannot reverse it. Low progesterone levels in early pregnancy are the result rather than the cause of miscarriage.'

After the egg has been fertilised, the womb (endometrium) lining will also stay thick where the embryo will implant and develop. If the womb lining is inadequate, then the embryo will not 'hold on' and a miscarriage will occur. It is possible to have good levels of progesterone and yet have a thin womb lining, perhaps because the womb lining is not responding to the levels of progesterone. Other doctors, however, do give progesterone to women with a history of recurrent miscarriages and they have gone on to have a successful pregnancy.

Ultrasound can also be useful for those women with a history of recurrent miscarriages, as it can often pick up an indication of corpus luteum failure before any drop in progesterone level is seen in the blood. This is where the use of progesterone can be beneficial.

There are so many factors that govern the efficient functioning of the cycle that it is not always easy to identify cause and effect. Every part of the cycle is dependent on what went before so we may not be able to 'fix' problems in the second half of the cycle without looking at what has gone wrong in the first half. By going back to the basic foundations of health and getting yourself back into balance, you have a much better chance of maintaining a pregnancy without the need for hormones or other drugs.

Auto-immune Disorders

These disorders occur when a woman produces antibodies directly against her own cells. The antibodies are thought to cause blood clots in the placenta, preventing the baby getting enough nutrients and blood. Treatment involves drugs that thin the blood, like aspirin and heparin.

An auto-immune condition called systemic lupus erythematosis (SLE) causes chronic inflammation which can affect many systems of the body. One of the world's leading experts in this disorder is Professor Graham Hughes, Head of the Lupus Arthritis Research Unit at St Thomas's Hospital in London. His original investigations showed that many lupus sufferers also had a blood clotting syndrome which can be detected through the presence of antiphospholipid antibodies in the blood. Lupus sufferers get pregnant easily but have a high rate of miscarriages. This syndrome has now been called Hughes Syndrome. It is like having 'sticky blood', which can trigger a miscarriage by causing blood clots to form in the placenta. It is also thought that these antibodies can directly attack the cells of the placenta, making implantation difficult. Hughes Syndrome can sometimes be found in women who do not have symptoms of SLE but are having recurrent miscarriages.

The two main antiphospholipid antibodies that need to be tested for are lupus anticoagulant and anticardiolipin antibodies. Professor Lesley Regan, of the Recurrent Miscarriage Clinic at St Mary's Hospital in London, has pioneered this work on antiphospholipid antibodies and miscarriages. She makes it clear that women need to have a number of tests to determine whether they have positive antibodies, as fluctuations can occur. You can also get false positive readings and so she recommends that women should test positive on at least two occasions, with each test performed at least eight weeks apart.

The treatment of choice for 'sticky blood' is aspirin. This has been a surprise because previous studies have linked taking aspirin in pregnancy with children's heart disease, brain malformations and cleft palates. Very heavy doses have been blamed for preventing normal growth of the lungs and 'blue baby syndrome'. The difference is that in this treatment the aspirin dose is low – only 76mg daily. The aspirin is given prior to conception and as soon as the woman finds out she is pregnant she is also given the anticoagulant drug heparin.

Trials at St Mary's have shown that the combination of aspirin and heparin works more effectively than just aspirin alone. As with any drug treatment, one has to weigh up the benefits against the risks: it has been reported that women taking heparin during pregnancy may have an increased risk of osteoporosis (thinning of the bones) and they will need to be monitored. Further larger studies are needed in order to confirm the miscarriage benefits of aspirin and heparin.

Another possibility, instead of either aspirin or heparin, is to use vitamin E. This vitamin can help thin the blood and prevent clots. Aspirin is often recommended for people who are at risk of heart attacks, in order to keep their blood thin and reduce the possibility of a clot. Yet a study published in the *Lancet* in 1996 found that taking a daily dose of vitamin E reduced the risk of having a heart attack by an astonishing 75 per cent.[204] The scientists heading this study commented that the results were even more 'exciting than aspirin'.

Unfortunately a number of women are now being given aspirin, as a 'just in case' measure, without any of the blood tests showing positive to the blood clotting factor.

The recommended dose of vitamin E should be around 400iu and you should buy the natural form of this vitamin, d-alpha tocopherol (see Chapter 10).

Immunotherapy

Some clinics have used a treatment called immunotherapy to stop miscarriages where there may have been several in a row. This treatment is based on the theory that a woman needs to produce special blocking antibodies to prevent her body rejecting the baby whose cells are different from her own. Normally our bodies try to reject any cells that are not ours and yet 50 per cent of a baby's cells are the partner's. This treatment is highly controversial. If the theory is right you may wonder why our bodies don't just reject the sperm to begin with, as they would any foreign object.

It is thought that the immune system's normal level of activity has to reduce slightly in order to 'accept' the growing baby. This reduction in immune activity is one reason why women who have rheumatoid arthritis can lose all their symptoms while pregnant. Rheumatoid arthritis is an inflammatory disorder with an auto-immune component and so benefits from a 'quieter' immune system. Immunotherapy treatment works like a vaccine and involves injecting the woman with her partner's blood to help her produce these antibodies. There have been doubts as to whether the treatment actually works and concern that it may cause sterility in some women, along with other problems such as transfusion reactions and hepatitis.

Incompetent Cervix

In a healthy pregnancy the neck of the womb (the cervix) remains closed until near the birth. However, when the cervix is incompetent the neck of the womb painlessly dilates without contractions, resulting in miscarriage or premature birth. The condition may be congenital (i.e. the woman was born with it) or may be the result of a previous pregnancy. With an incompetent cervix, the miscarriage is usually later – often into the second trimester of pregnancy. The usual treatment is to hold the cervix together with a stitch. Some doctors put the stitch in before conception, others in early pregnancy, and others only after the third month. The diagnosis for this condition is difficult and the research has not led to any clear-cut conclusions as to how beneficial the stitch really is. Obviously if it is inserted too early it could stop nature miscarrying an abnormal baby.

Anatomical abnormalities

An unusually shaped womb may cause problems with implantation. Some women can be born with problems, such as a double uterus (womb), and yet can go on to have healthy pregnancies, while the same condition in others can cause them to miscarry. Surgery is a possibility if your womb is abnormal.

Abnormal Sperm

Because it is the woman who miscarries, greater emphasis has been placed on looking at problems in the female reproductive system. But if you keep miscarrying when nothing can be found wrong it is logical to wonder if the problem might be with your partner's sperm instead. Early studies have shown that there is an increased risk of miscarriage where there are sperm abnormalities.[205] So it really is important that both the man and woman get themselves into optimum health before conception.

Smoking

A study published in the *British Journal of Cancer* showed that men who smoke, while their partner doesn't, run the risk of fathering children who develop cancers such as leukaemia and brain tumours.[206] The theory is that chemicals in tobacco smoke can damage the DNA in the sperm. Taking this one step further, it's easy to see that any changes in DNA in the sperm could lead to a possible increase in miscarriage rate. DNA damage cannot be picked up in a normal semen analysis so this problem would not be seen during routine fertility investigations.

Quite apart from the possible increase in abnormalities in babies of women who smoke during pregnancy (see Chapter 8), there is also an increased risk of miscarriages.[207]

Another study, by Professor Jane Golding of the Royal Hospital for Children in Bristol, highlighted how our own actions can affect the next generation. Jane Golding looked at daughters who didn't smoke but whose mothers had smoked. The daughters subsequently suffered a significantly increased risk of miscarriages.[208]

Alcohol

Chapter 8 discussed the direct effects of alcohol on fertility and pregnancy but it is important to remember the enormous impact this substance can have on the risk of miscarriages. It is universally acknowledged that alcohol can alter a man's sperm count and cause an increase in abnormal sperm.[209] Therefore, it follows that if an abnormal sperm fertilises an egg, nature will try to 'get rid' of that embryo because it is working on 'survival of the fittest'.

Alcohol is a substance that is known to cause mutations. For example, studies have shown that alcohol given to female mice immediately after mating caused severe damage to the chromosomes of one-fifth to one-sixth of the embryos.[210] This resulted in a higher percentage of miscarriages or death shortly after birth. Chromosomal damage is a recognised cause of miscarriage.

Research has also shown a strong relationship between alcohol and miscarriages. A 1977 study found that women who have a drink every day have a risk of miscarriage 2.5 times higher than non-drinkers.[211] In this same study they found that if the woman was a drinker and a smoker her risk of having a miscarriage increased by up to four times.

The conclusion, from a number of the studies on women, is that even moderate alcohol consumption works as a reproductive toxin and as such increases the risk of a miscarriage.[212]

Caffeine

Caffeine is a stimulant and could therefore be classed as a 'drug'. It has an adverse effect on fertility (see page 51) but it can also cause problems once a woman is pregnant.

In a study of 2967 pregnant women, carried out by the Department of Epidemiology and Public Health at Yale University School of Medicine, the researchers found that drinking three or more cups of tea or coffee a day was associated with an increased risk of miscarriage.[213] Other research has shown that caffeine during pregnancy can increase the probability of chromosomal abnormality which could lead to a miscarriage.[214]

Since 1980 the US Food and Drug Administration has advised pregnant women to minimise their caffeine intake, citing the dangers of possible miscarriages or having a mentally retarded baby. Some studies suggest that there is a doubly increased risk of foetal loss when as little as one to three cups of coffee are consumed a day. So the logical advice is to err on the side of caution and avoid caffeine altogether, especially if you have a history of recurrent miscarriages.[215]

Even decaffeinated coffee has been linked to an increased risk of miscarriage,[216] since there is still some caffeine left even after decaffeination. Moreover, decaffeinated coffee contains two other stimulants, theobromine and theophylline, which are not removed when the coffee is decaffeinated. Also most decaffeinated coffee has been decaffeinated by a chemical which can remain in the product.

An important point to remember is that caffeine comes in many other forms besides tea and coffee. It is there in colas and other soft drinks, as well as chocolate, and pain-relieving medication, such as headache remedies.

Selenium Deficiency

Selenium is a powerful antioxidant which may help prevent DNA damage. Researchers have found that those women who miscarry have low levels of selenium in their blood compared to women who don't miscarry.[217]

Radiation

Visual Display Units (VDUs) on computers emit non-ionising radiation, as indeed do microwaves, televisions, electric blankets, mobile phones and other electrical appliances. A number of studies have looked at the effects on women who work in front of computers, but the results are not conclusive.

Concerns about VDUs originated in Canada. In 1980, it was reported that a large number of birth defects were present in one group of VDU operators.[218] Another study in 1984 showed that, out of 55 pregnancies of VDU users, 14.5 per cent ended in miscarriage, as compared to 5.3 per cent in non-VDU users. A further 22 per cent of the pregnancies had resulted in a malformation, compared to 11 per cent in non-VDU user. And 6.7 per cent had suffered a stillbirth, as compared to only 1 per cent in the other group.[219] The Royal College of Obstetricians and Gynaecologists in the UK suggests that VDUs are not a hazard.

With the evidence as it stands at present, I personally feel it is sensible to limit time on VDUs during pregnancy. This is not only because of the possibility of unknown risk factors but also because working for long, uninterrupted periods in front of VDUs is stressful and can cause other symptoms such as headaches, nausea, fatigue, insomnia and menstrual disturbances.[221] There is good evidence to show that stress in some women can stop them ovulating,[221] and may also have adverse effects during pregnancy.

Other sources of radiation, such as X-rays and microwave ovens, are covered in Chapters 4, 5 and 13. If a woman is going for an X-ray she is usually asked to do it in the first half of the cycle so that she cannot be pregnant without knowing it.

Conclusion

If you look objectively at the many hormones that govern your reproductive cycle, you can see how they must all work together in order to conceive healthy babies. Much fertility treatment involves boosting this or that hormone – often by excessive amounts – to 'trick' the body. In the case of miscarriages, the doctors may suspect an inadequate level of proges-terone, or too high a level of LH, and so use drugs to try to rectify the imbalance. But, like any drug, the treatment will have its own side-effects and repercussions. On the other hand, by giving your body the right nutrients, minimising environmental hazards, and getting into optimum health, you and your partner can do a great deal to help prevent another miscarriage.

SECTION 6

PUTTING IT ALL
INTO PRACTICE

❀

So you've read the information in this book and feel that it makes sense. Now you want to put it all into practice. What do you do first? How do you go about getting the best of both the medical and complementary worlds?

You may have been trying to conceive for a while and not be sure what to do next. Or you may have already been down the path of fertility investigations and want to know what else can be done. Couples who come and see me often remark that nobody else has pulled all the strands together – they feel they need to follow a logically structured plan that includes all the factors that could affect their fertility. This is what my Four-Month Preconception Plan offers.

I am suggesting that you follow this Four-Month Plan and do *not* try to conceive within that time. Why? Because when you follow the plan your fertility will start to increase. Time and time again, a couple will say 'we have been trying for six years so it's not going to happen in the next four months' and yet it does. But the risk is that, if you conceive before everything is back to optimum levels, you may increase the chance of a miscarriage.

CHAPTER 21

The Four-Month Preconception Plan

Following the Four-Month Preconception Plan means:

1. eating a healthy diet
2. checking and correcting your nutritional status
3. adopting a healthy lifestyle
4. being screened for infections
5. avoiding environmental hazards
6. timing your fertility investigations

1 Eating a Healthy Diet

This is the most important step because good nutrition is the foundation on which your health is built and the key to increasing your chances of conceiving. Look at what you are eating and drinking, buy organic food where possible, eat a good variety of food (including fish, nuts, seeds, fresh fruit and vegetables), and read labels to reduce or eliminate the amount of chemicals, additives and preservatives going into your body. It's also important to get your weight back into the normal range, if you are underweight or overweight.

Carry on eating well over the four months and until you become pregnant, and through the pregnancy itself.

2 Checking and Correcting Your Nutritional Status

Where possible, at the very beginning of the Four-Month Plan, you should go to a nutritional therapist (see Useful Addresses). Preferably choose one with experience in fertility and have a full assessment of your vitamin and mineral deficiencies. You will also be checked to see whether you have high levels of heavy toxic metals, such as lead, mercury and cadmium. You will then be given a programme of food supplements for four months to correct any deficiencies and to lower any toxic metals. At the end of the four months the assessment should be repeated, to make sure that the nutrients have been absorbed and the levels are back to normal. Once back to normal, you will be given a maintenance programme to stay on until you conceive.

If you are worried about the cost, bear in mind that IVF treatment is expensive (often in the region of £2,000–3,000 per treatment cycle). The investment in seeing a nutritional therapist, together with taking a programme of food supplements, therefore is minimal in comparison and may mean you avoid the IVF altogether. If you still need IVF treatment, the investment is still worthwhile because it increases the chance of it working.

For those who can't get to see a nutritional therapist, I have devised a proposed supplement programme. Normally the programme would be personalised for you and your partner and would depend on what deficiencies you each had, but here you are both taking almost the same supplements.

Supplement Programme

Take:

- a multivitamin and mineral designed for pregnancy
- zinc citrate or amino acid chelate (total of 30mg of zinc a day, including what is in the multivitamin and mineral)
- 1000mg linseed (or flax oil) a day
- 1000mg vitamin C a day

If your partner has a low sperm count or motility he needs to add 1,000mg of L-arginine a day to this programme for sperm health and 300–400ius a day of vitamin E to help fertilisation.

To make this programme simpler I have formulated two supplements called Fertility Plus for Women and Fertility Plus for Men.

Fertility Plus for Women contains those nutrients known to help with fertility and you would only need to add the linseed oil and vitamin C. It is designed to provide the nutrients needed leading up to and during pregnancy. It contains the required amount of folic acid (400mcg a day) so you don't need to take a separate folic acid supplement. It also includes a safe amount of vitamin A that you can take during pregnancy.

Fertility Plus for Men contains those nutrients which are helpful for men trying to conceive, including L-arginine, L-carnitine and also vitamin E.

If you have difficulty getting Fertility Plus call the phone number on page 242 and they can be sent to you.

If you are following this Four-Month Plan without being nutritionally tested then stay on the above supplement programme not just for the four months but until you conceive.

3 Adopting a Healthy Lifestyle

Look at your lifestyle, including alcohol, smoking and street drugs, and make sure you and your partner eliminate these during the four months. Remember, it takes around three months for a man to produce a new batch of sperm so by the end of the Four-Month Plan these new healthy, mobile sperm will have a much greater chance of fertilising your egg. It also takes three months for your egg to start from a group of follicles, and then to be selected as the egg that is released on the cycle.

Eliminate any unnecessary over-the-counter drugs both of you may be taking. You should also ask your doctor whether any prescribed medication you may be taking could be affecting your fertility and whether there are alternatives to these drugs.

Get your partner to buy looser underwear and trousers and take showers instead of hot baths. If he sits down all day, suggest he thinks about taking breaks and walking around, especially if he is sitting down driving in a hot vehicle.

4 Being Screened for Infections

Make sure that both you and your partner are checked for any genito-urinary infections (GUIs). This is especially important before you embark on any fertility testing because, if an infection is present, certain investigations via the vagina could push the infection higher up inside the body.

This step is also crucial if you have had a previous miscarriage, just to rule out the possibility that an infection was not the cause.

Your GP may organise this screen for you or you can go to the GUI clinic at your local hospital (they will not be able to test all those on the list in Chapter 17). Both you and your partner should be tested.

At the moment, in my opinion, not enough emphasis is placed on this kind of testing. If you have any problems organising these checks then my contact details are at the back of the book (see page 242).

If an infection shows up, you and/or your partner will be treated. You should then have a re-test to make sure the infection has cleared up.

Most infections will require treatment with an antibiotic. This is not ideal, and in complementary medicine it is usual to try to avoid the use of antibiotics. In this situation, however, the infection may be long-standing and it must be cleared up fairly quickly because it may be stopping you conceiving. Antibiotics wipe out the infection but they will also wipe out the beneficial bacteria which live in the gut, leaving you prone to thrush. So, as soon as you have finished the course of antibiotics, you need to take a good probiotic (the opposite of an antibiotic which helps to re-colonise the gut flora). Use:

- BioCare's Replete – one sachet per day for seven days
- Then go on to BioCare's Bio-acidophilus for one month

5 Avoiding Environmental Hazards

Think about your environment. Could your occupation or your partner's be affecting fertility (e.g. farming with pesticides, hairdressing with dye, hairspray, etc, or painting). And can you do anything to reduce the problem?

In your home, can you limit the amount of chemicals used? For example, can you avoid using pesticides in the garden, and flea sprays in the house? If you are decorating the house, finish the work before you begin the Four-Month Plan.

6 Timing Your Fertility Investigations

Now you have put into place a good food supplement programme, looked at your diet and your environment and know that you are free from infections. The next step is that of fertility investigations.

However, the speed with which you take this next step depends on a number of factors and I would like to suggest a guide for assessing this.

If You Have Been Trying to Conceive for Six Months

If you have been trying for six months and are under the age of 35, follow steps 1–5 (above) for four months. At the end of the four months, try to conceive for six months on your own before embarking on any fertility investigations.

If you have been trying for six months and are over 35, follow steps 1–5 but start on the fertility investigations during the four months. If you are given a diagnosis of unexplained infertility, then try for six months on your own before going for medical treatment.

If You Have Been Trying to Conceive for 12 Months or More

If you are under the age of 35, follow steps 1–5 over the four-month period. Then try on your own for six months before embarking on fertility tests.

If you are over 35, follow steps 1–5 for four months and during that four months go for fertility checks. If you get a diagnosis of unexplained infertility, try for six months on your own before you go for treatment.

Taking Age into Account

Because fertility declines with age, if you are over 35 you urgently need to know your fertility status. For example, if you are 40 and you have followed the plan for four months, waited another six months to try and then found out you've got blocked fallopian tubes you are going to need IVF treatment. In that situation it is better to know sooner rather than later so a decision can be made.

If You are Going to Have Assisted Conception

If you are told that IVF (or ICSI) is your best option then you should still take the time to follow the Four-Month Preconception Plan first. Those four months are so crucial, no matter what age you are. You want you and your partner to be in optimum health before you go for the IVF treatment, to give it the best chance of working. You want to produce good-quality eggs that will be fertilised easily with good-quality sperm, and you want your body to be as healthy as possible to increase the possibility of those fertilised eggs implanting when they are put back and staying there.

Making an Informed Decision

If you are embarking on fertility investigations you want to get maximum information in minimum time, especially if you are over the age of 35. This enables you to make an informed decision. Essentially, you want to know:

- Is ovulation taking place?
- Are your hormone levels normal, at the beginning and end of the cycle?
- Are your fallopian tubes clear (patent)?
- Once you ovulate, is your womb lining thick enough for a fertilised egg to implant?
- Could any other problem, such as endometriosis, be stopping you conceiving?
- Is your partner's sperm count good and are a high percentage of the sperm motile and normal?

To get this amount of information fairly quickly, you will probably need to go to a private clinic. But it is well worth it and the consultation time is usually longer, allowing you more time to ask questions.

The ideal situation is a clinic which takes a holistic approach to infertility and where medical tests and treatment are timed to coordinate with nutritional medicine. (I know of only one clinic where this approach is used and that is Reproductive Healthcare in London where I work – see page 228)

At the End of the Four Months

Have your vitamins, minerals and heavy toxic metal levels re-assessed to make sure they are back to normal. You will then be given a maintenance programme of supplements to keep the levels up while you try to conceive or go through medical treatment, depending on your situation.

Conclusion

Critics of nutritional therapy often claim that people who go to a nutritional therapist and get results are only feeling better because of a placebo effect. For instance, if somebody goes to see a nutritional therapist because they have a skin problem and is given a programme of supplements, critics say that the person could still believe their skin condition was better even if the supplements given were dummy pills.

Infertility, however, is very different. You either have a baby or you don't. Your skin can feel a little bit better but you cannot be a little bit pregnant. The result is not subjective. When you see, as I do, couples who have been trying to conceive for up to ten years conceive, or couples who have had five miscarriages get pregnant and have a healthy baby after making simple lifestyle changes, there is no doubting the results.

Others claim that it is the fact that a nutritional therapist spends time listening to a couple (usually an hour for the first consultation) that makes the difference. If it is that simple, why aren't doctors just increasing their consultation time?

The other point is, what have you got to lose by following this plan? In fact, you have everything to gain. Not only will your health improve but you will also increase your chances of conceiving, having a healthy pregnancy and giving birth to a healthy baby. And, based on what scientists are now finding out about the importance of foetal programming and the environment in the womb, you are helping to give your baby long-term health right through to adulthood.

LOOKING AFTER YOUR HEALTH DURING PREGNANCY

❊

You should be feeling on top of the world. Not only are you pregnant at last but, because you have been following the plan these past months, you and your partner are probably feeling healthier than you have for years. You now want to prepare for a comfortable pregnancy and the safe delivery of a healthy baby.

I hope that you can now see for yourselves how absolutely crucial nutrition has been in achieving your pregnancy. So just imagine its importance for the development of your baby. In the early weeks and months of pregnancy the baby's cells divide and multiply rapidly and its organs are formed. So I cannot stress too much the importance of maintaining your nutritional programme during pregnancy.

You may think that babies in the womb are insulated in a protective environment – that this is nature's way of protecting the next generation. But this is only true up to a point. More and more research is showing that what happens to an expectant mother – what she eats or doesn't eat, for instance – has a profound effect on her baby's health both now and in the future.

Fortunately, following the Four-Month Preconception Plan not only helps you conceive. It also reduces the risk of having a baby which is underweight, premature, or born with malformations.

What You Should Do Now

If you are taking herbal supplements you should stop these as soon as you think you may be pregnant. If you are seeing a nutritional therapist you will be given a supplement maintenance programme. If you are following the recommendations in this book without professional advice you can just carry on taking the same supplements. Obviously your partner can stop if he wishes – his job is now over as far as conception is concerned.

It is vital that you continue to have a good level of nutrition all the way through your pregnancy. There is evidence that vitamin supplements can prevent one of the most dangerous conditions that can occur in pregnancy, pre-eclampsia, which can be fatal for mother and child. This condition is believed to be linked to poor nutrition and the symptoms are high blood pressure, swelling in the hands and feet, and protein in the urine. It has been found that the placenta and the white blood cells of women with pre-eclampsia produce free radicals.

In 1999 the *Lancet* published the results of the first trial to see if vitamin supplements were effective in preventing pre-eclampsia.[223] Half a group of pregnant women, some with a history of the condition and others with an abnormal blood flow to the placenta, were given vitamin E and vitamin C supplements. The other half were given a placebo. The group who took the vitamins had a 76 per cent reduction in pre-eclampsia, compared to those taking the placebo. At least four other studies over the last few years have confirmed the link between low levels of antioxidants and a higher risk of pre-eclampsia. And other research has shown that women with the lowest levels of Omega 3 fatty acids (which come from fish and linseeds) are more likely to have pre-eclampsia.[224] Both vitamin E and Omega 3 essential oils help to prevent blood clotting and abnormal blood flow to the placenta.

This is why it is so important to continue with a good level of nutrition all the way through pregnancy as well as in the preconception period. It can prevent so many problems occurring – and scientists are only just finding out the full impact of these nutrients, or their deficiencies, on the mother and developing baby.

CHAPTER 22

Eating Well

Those who are sceptical about the importance of nutrition in preconceptual care argue that there are many cultures where the women are living through famine and yet we see them on the television with babies. They conclude that the lack of nourishment is not affecting their fertility.

However, studies have shown that in fact the babies are not born to the most undernourished women (as they are infertile) but to those whose intake is marginal, and the unfortunate outcome is sick babies. A number of studies have looked at fertility and what happens to babies when food is in short supply. During the short but terrible Dutch famine of 1944–5, right at the end of the Second World War,[225] it was found that the timing of malnutrition was crucial. Women who conceived or were in the early part of their pregnancy when the famine struck had many more babies who died around the time of birth than women who were in the later part of a pregnancy when the food shortages happened.[226]

This finding ties in with those on the effects of alcohol during pregnancy (see page 74) which is more damaging in the first 12 weeks. During the Dutch food shortage half the women of childbearing age lost their periods (i.e. became temporarily infertile). There was also an increase in stillbirths for those babies conceived during the food shortage.

Appallingly, there was also an increase in malformations among the babies born nine months after the Dutch hunger winter. These babies were conceived during the worst of the food shortage, and the impact seemed to continue in those women who conceived four months *after* the shortage was over. The implication is that they were still suffering the effects of malnutrition. This provides further evidence to support having a Four-Month Preconception Plan, to get the maximum benefit for fertility and the health of the baby.

Nature is extremely clever. At a time of food shortage, when the woman does not even have enough nutrients to nourish itself, it stands to reason that she cannot nourish a baby properly. So, in extreme cases of famine, the body shuts down its reproductive function, in order to avoid risking the baby's health. The reproductive system is the only system we do not need to survive. In a time of literally life and death, the body channels its resources away from the reproductive system to other areas of greater need. As soon as the food supply is plentiful, periods return and fertility is often restored as soon as the first month, but an epidemic of miscarriages can often then follow.[227]

Poor maternal nutrition during the most sensitive period of the baby's development may produce lifelong changes in physiology and structure. And the most rapid cell division is taking place before most women know they are pregnant. The brain, heart and other major organs develop in the first month. When the placenta takes over, around the twelfth week of pregnancy, it can extract the nutrients from the mother's blood for the baby. So, in the later stages of pregnancy, the mother could be nutritionally defi- cient and yet the baby would not suffer, unless the mother was severely malnourished. In mothers who subsequently gave birth to low birthweight babies, 43 out of 44 nutrients measured in the mothers were significantly below those of mothers whose babies fell in the normal range.[228]

Unfortunately, and astonishingly, the UK ranks alongside Albania as having one of the worst statistics in Europe for producing seriously under- weight babies according to the World Health Organisation. As many as 7 per cent of babies in England and Wales are classed as 'low birthweight', which puts them more at risk of stillbirth, mental handicap, dying within a month, blindness, deafness, cerebral palsy and autism. Within Europe, only Hungary (9 per cent) and Poland (8 per cent) have worst statistics than us.

Low Birthweight

Low birthweight is classed as any baby weighing under 2.5kg (5.5lb) at birth. In my mother's generation it was desirable to have a large baby because they were considered to be stronger. In baby competitions of that era, babies that won first prize were usually bigger and classed as 'bonny babies'. The trend then moved to the opposite extreme – women felt that a smaller baby looked cuter and they also thought that a smaller baby would mean an easier labour.

However, pioneering work by Professor David Barker has shown that what we weigh at birth can have an immense effect on our health later on in life. Low birthweight has been linked to an increased risk of high blood pressure,[229] a higher risk of coronary heart disease,[230] and a greater risk of non-insulin dependent diabetes.[231]

As David Barker says, 'Research suggests that coronary heart disease and stroke and the associated conditions, hypertension [high blood pressure] and non-insulin dependent diabetes, originate through impaired growth and development during foetal life and infancy.'

A 1997 study looked at women who were born with low birthweights. The scientists then monitored the same women through puberty and adolescence, and found that they started their periods about three to six months later than average. When they became pregnant, the course of pregnancy and delivery was within the normal range but their chance of giving birth to a low birthweight baby was double that of other women.[232] This is why preconception care, and what you do once you are pregnant, is so important.

The World Health Organisation uses two markers for the health of any nation: birthweight and longevity. In the UK 54,000 low birthweight babies are born each year and the incidence has not changed in 30 years.

These consequences of low birthweight affect the babies throughout their lives and it is now suggested that there is a link between weight at birth and asthma. Researchers from a number of London hospitals found that low birthweight was a risk factor for asthma by the age of 26. The incidence of asthma among adults fell as birthweight increased.

Nutrition plays a key role in helping you to get pregnant and then having a healthy pregnancy and a healthy baby. All the recommendations in this book for preconception care are just as important once you are pregnant, including the continued use of food supplements.

As Isobel Jennings says in her book *Vitamins in Endocrine Metabolism*, 'It seems that much more could be done in the field of preventative medicine to cut down the large numbers of preventable congenital defects. In human foetal development, most abnormalities are established by the eighth to the tenth week of gestation. This means of course that the most important period for nutritional care occurs in the few weeks before and immediately after conception.'[233]

A few years ago, Scandinavian doctors linked diets rich in fish with a decrease in premature births. They felt that three fish meals a week would be enough not only to reduce premature births but also to produce a good weight baby.

Foetal Programming

Scientists used to think that adult illnesses (like heart disease, breast cancer, diabetes and obesity) were either the direct result of what we have inherited through our genes or were due to unhealthy living patterns. Current research, however, suggests instead that we are programmed to be susceptible to these illnesses depending on what we were exposed to in the womb. This concept – that the diseases of adult life could be connected to conditions in the womb – is called foetal programming.

The research by Professor David Barker mentioned earlier (which showed the link between our birthweight and the possibility of heart problems) is just one aspect of this programming. It seems that whatever conditions in the womb stunt the baby's growth also increases their risk of cardiovascular disease. Scientists are now taking this research further by looking at other traits which may be influenced in the womb, such as high cholesterol, obesity, diabetes, breast cancer, mental illness and intelligence.

This new science of foetal programming is even causing a rethink of genetic influences. For instance, it has always been thought that identical twins are more likely to share a similar characteristic because this characteristic was controlled by their genes. But identical twins also share the same conditions in the womb so could other factors be at work?

Recent research, published in the *American Journal of Clinical Nutrition*, monitored the daughters born to those women who were pregnant during the Dutch famine of 1944–45 (see page 196). They found that those women whose mothers were malnourished during the early stages of pregnancy because of the famine had a significantly greater chance of being obese at the age of 50. If the mothers had been starved *after* the first four months of their pregnancy there was no difference in the Body Mass Index (see page 58) for these daughters, compared with an average cross-section of similar age. The researchers concluded that the obesity developed as a result of permanent changes 'fixed' in the womb, rather than as the result of the usual lifestyle factors.

Further findings from this research also suggest that the children of the women who were pregnant during the famine have a greater risk of developing late-onset diabetes.

Professor Barker is suggesting that, because different issues in the foetus have different critical periods of development, the timing of an effect on a woman is crucial. The converse is also true. If we nourish the baby in the womb as healthily as possible we can lessen the risk of the child developing future illnesses.

This does not mean that we have no control over our health as adults. But it may put us more at risk of developing a certain problem like heart disease later on in life, requiring us to be more careful about our diet, exercise, etc. But, more importantly, this research shows that certain adult illnesses could be prevented if we concentrated on making the environment in the womb as healthy as possible.

CHAPTER 23

Staying Off Alcohol and Cigarettes

Alcohol

You may be told by your doctor not to drink during the first three months of pregnancy but it is fine after that as long as it's only one or two glasses now and again. However, unfortunately, we now know that even a little bit can be too much. During the first 12 weeks, the highest rate of cell division takes place and all the major organs are formed, so there is more risk if a toxin like alcohol gets to the baby then. After the third month the baby grows and matures. This period is important because, even though the baby is fully formed, his or her organs cannot function on their own yet. As well as the heart and lungs the brain is also maturing. It is the brain that can be vulnerable to damage after the first 12 weeks.

It has been known for centuries that drinking during pregnancy can cause problems with the health of the baby. In the 1720s 'gin epidemic', the Royal College of Physicians stated that parental drinking was a cause of 'weak, feeble and distempered children'.[234]

Alcohol is classed as a teratogen (an agent or drug that can cause malformation of an embryo or foetus). Professor David Smith from Washington points out that 'there is no known teratogen yet studied in man which clearly shows a threshold effect where the substance is quite safe to a particular level, beyond which it is teratogenic'.[235] In effect, he is saying that the experts cannot say that one glass a week would be fine but two glasses are not. As the World Health Organisation states, 'no alcohol during pregnancy is the only safe limit'.

By day 36 of pregnancy, the neural tube of the embryo opens and a rudimentary system is formed. If a teratogenic substance like alcohol is drunk at this most crucial time, it can result in various malformations in the newborn (e.g. defective heart and muscular skeletal abnormalities).

Remember that you will be two weeks pregnant before you know you are. You only know that you might be pregnant when your period is late.

However, although the first three months are the most critical, the teratogenic effects of alcohol continue throughout pregnancy, affecting, at the later stages, brain development and function, in particular. Low birthweight and congenital abnormalities have all been linked to the teratogenic effect, with the probability of twice the risk of abnormalities.[236]

The placenta does not act as a barrier. Alcohol is a low molecular substance which is quite capable of crossing the placenta and entering the baby. It does not take a mathematician to work out that, in relative terms, a dose of alcohol must have a much more profound effect on a minute developing embryo than on the much larger mother.

Foetal Alcohol Syndrome

In its most extreme form, a mother's alcohol consumption can cause Foetal Alcohol Syndrome (FAS).[237] The characteristics of this syndrome include abnormalities of growth, craniofacial, musculoskeletal, cardiac, nervous system and neuro-developmental delay or mental deficiency, with an average IQ of 65. Babies born with Foetal Alcohol Syndrome will look visibly different from other babies. They may have reduced weight, length and head circumference compared to healthy babies and may be labelled as 'failing to thrive'. The nasal bridge can be poorly formed and the baby may have large ears which are simply formed. They may also have a cleft palate. Limb defects are also common, including such problems as congenital hip dislocations. Congenital heart disease is also a concern. As with any drug, the newborn baby may display signs of withdrawal symptoms, such as restlessness, and being fretful and tremulous.

Foetal Alcohol Effects

It is now recognised that some children do not bear the severe physical characteristics of FAS but still have subtle mental or behavioural difficulties caused by being exposed to alcohol in the womb. These characteristics have been identified as Foetal Alcohol Effects.[238] And they are produced merely by 'social drinking'.

One study looked at the effect of consuming two or more drinks most days during the pregnancy or binge drinking (drinking five or more drinks in one go, at a party for example) before the mother realised she was pregnant. The babies born from these mothers were followed over seven years to see how they progressed. From the beginning, the babies had a lower than average birthweight and were more jittery. They had difficulty establishing a good sucking pattern and had disrupted sleep patterns. From eight months, their co-ordination was not good and they still had disrupted sleep patterns.

A follow-up study at seven years old showed that those children whose mothers had been drinking two or more drinks a day were seven points lower in their IQ scores than the average seven-year-old. Children of mothers who had been binge drinking before they realised they were pregnant were approximately one to three months behind in reading and arithmetic. Other tests from this study showed a poor attention span, problems with memory and negative behaviour patterns.[239]

In fact, they had some of the classic symptoms of hyperactivity, now called attention deficit hyperactive disorder (ADHD). Cause and effect can be so difficult to pinpoint when results may be present seven years after the actual cause. But, instead of focusing attention on drugs such as Ritalin to control hyperactivity, maybe funding should be ploughed into preventative measures which could be as simple as asking women not to drink at all during pregnancy.

Alcohol is also a diuretic so it increases the urinary excretion of valuable vitamins and minerals. Zinc, a very important mineral during pregnancy, is depleted with alcohol consumption,[240] and studies show that when zinc levels are reduced, low birthweight and foetal malformations can follow.[241] Folic acid deficiency can also result from the diuretic effect of alcohol and this is the nutrient known to help prevent spina bifida.[242]

Clearly, alcohol is a toxin and there is no limit below which it is safe. In this situation it is definitely not the case that 'a little won't harm' and I cannot emphasise too strongly how important eliminating alcohol is to the health of your baby.

Smoking

There is so much information out there about the risks you run of getting lung cancer, emphysema and other diseases if you smoke. Thankfully, many people are now aware of the detrimental effects of smoking when a woman is pregnant.

Tobacco smoke contains more than 4,000 compounds and these pass directly into the foetal blood supply. These chemicals have different effects on the developing baby:

- **Nicotine** causes the foetal heart rate to accelerate. It also decreases blood flow to the placenta and can affect placental amino acid uptake, causing retarded growth of the baby.

- **Carbon monoxide** affects foetal blood flow to the brain, heart and adrenal glands and can affect brain DNA and protein synthesis.

- **Polycyclic aromatic hydrocarbons** are mutagens and carcinogens and can interfere with placental hormone activity.

- **Cyanide** can cause retarded infant growth.

No less than 45 studies have confirmed that smoking is a major cause of low birthweight.[243]

Lack of oxygen to the developing baby (foetal hypoxia), caused by cigarette smoking during pregnancy, also leads to a higher risk of prematurity and congenital abnormalities, as shown by numerous studies.[244]

Cadmium is an inorganic poison present in smoke which becomes concentrated in the placenta. It is classed, like alcohol, as a teratogen, and interferes with the utilisation of many important minerals including zinc. Cadmium is also a poison to the baby. In conjunction with low zinc status, it has been associated with human stillbirth, underweight babies and various forms of congenital abnormalities.[245]

The rate of premature births for mothers who smoke 30 cigarettes a day is 33 per cent, compared to only 6 per cent for non-smoking mothers. Studies have found that smokers (both male and female) are more likely to have children with all types of congenital malformations (in particular cleft palate, hare lip, squints and deafness). Even if you don't smoke, but your partner smokes over 10 cigarettes a day, you are 2.5 times more likely to have a child with congenital malformations.

These substances should also be avoided during pregnancy and breast-feeding. If your partner insists on smoking he should not smoke in the house or when you are with him. Only 15 per cent of the smoke from a cigarette is inhaled; the rest goes into the air and will be inhaled by those near the smoker.[246]

Children of parents who smoke inhale amounts of nicotine equivalent to them actively smoking 60–150 cigarettes a year.[247] This results in an increased risk of asthma, chest infections, and ear, nose and throat infections for children. It is estimated that 50 children a day are admitted to hospital due to the effects of passive smoking.

Cot Death

Smoking mothers also put their babies at higher risk of Sudden Infant Death Syndrome (or cot death). Professor Jean Golding, of the Royal Hospital for Children in Bristol, found that, in comparison to a mother who doesn't smoke at all, mothers who smoke between one and two cigarettes a day are 80 per cent more likely to have a baby who suffers a cot death and those smoking more than 10 a day are nearly three times as likely to have such a death.[248]

Professor Golding also studied boys born to smoking mothers. These boys were significantly more likely to have undescended testes. So the effects of these toxins are literally being passed on from generation to generation and will have a long-term effect not only on the sexual development of a woman's own children but also on her grandchildren.

CHAPTER 24

Avoiding Infections, Drugs and Toxins

Infections

As we have seen (page 23), chlamydia can damage your fertility. And, once you are pregnant, it can cause other problems.

An infected pregnant woman can pass on chlamydia trachomatis to her baby during delivery, resulting in conjunctivitis, failure to thrive, gastro-enteritis and respiratory problems. It may also be a causal agent for otitis media ('glue ear'),[249] so it needs to be treated as soon as possible when diagnosed.

Toxins

Mercury

Mercury is a toxic metal found in dental fillings and there are concerns about its effects during pregnancy. One study demonstrated how quickly mercury passes from the mother to the baby. Pregnant sheep were fitted with 12 molars filled with amalgam (a mixture of mercury and other metals used in dentistry). These contained radioactive mercury so that the researchers could track the path of the mercury. As early as three days after putting in the fillings, mercury accumulation was seen in both the mother's and baby's blood and in the amniotic fluid. The mercury was also present in the baby's kidneys and liver, which showed higher mercury accumulation than the mother. After the birth of the lambs, the mercury continued to be transferred to the lambs via the milk, with the level in the milk testing eight times higher than in the mother's blood.

The Department of Health has suggested that pregnant women do not have mercury (amalgam) fillings during pregnancy. I would take that further and recommend that you avoid all dental work, if at all possible, during pregnancy.

Occupational Hazards

Many occupations pose a risk once the woman is pregnant. It has been found that pregnant women exposed to organic solvents have a 13-fold risk of having a baby with a serious congenital malformation. These solvents can be present in the printing, graphic design, clothing, textile and healthcare professions. The suspected solvents include hydrocarbons, phenols, trichloroethylene, xylene, vinyl chloride and acetone.[250]

Normal office equipment, such as photocopiers, fax machines, computers and laser printers, can produce high levels of ozone. It is worth keeping the office stocked with plants to keep the air as fresh as possible. Houseplants will stop the air becoming too dry, as well as absorbing a certain amount of radiation and acting as air purifiers.

You may be in a job that regularly exposes you to hazards and you will need to think about whether the risk can be minimised or whether you may have to change your occupation. Women exposed to pesticides can have miscarriages, stillbirths and babies with malformations.[251] This is why it is so important to think about your occupation and consider whether you have to make changes in order to protect yourself and your child.

Drugs

Street Drugs

The use of street drugs like marijuana and cocaine has increased steadily over the years. However, as well as their adverse effects on fertility, these drugs can also affect the development and health of the growing baby.

In animals, marijuana has been linked to stillbirths and malformations.[252] In general, it has similar effects to tobacco smoking such as low birthweight.

If women use cocaine once they are pregnant they are more likely to have a miscarriage, a stillbirth or a baby born with a malformation.[253]

The number of stillbirths increases in women who take heroin while they are pregnant, and the rate of prematurity goes up.[254] Also, babies born to mothers who have taken heroin and cocaine suffer withdrawal symptoms which can be severe.

The message has to be that these drugs need to be eliminated from your body at least four months before you try to conceive.

Medication

You should try to avoid taking any drugs while pregnant. If you are taking tranquillisers and sleeping pills, talk to your doctor about gradually coming off them and finding other ways to deal with the problem (such as relaxation techniques).

Even ordinary, over-the-counter drugs can have an effect on pregnancy. For instance, paracetamol and ibuprofen can inhibit the production of prostaglandins which are essential for the healthy development of the foetus.

Taking analgesics or painkillers – the kind you buy at the chemists and in the supermarket – has been shown to increase the risk of miscarriages,[255] and paracetamol has been linked to causing mutations in both animals and human cells.[256]

One kind of tranquilliser, called benzodiazepines (BZD), is often taken during pregnancy but could cause irreversible central nervous system and behavioural disorders. The UK drug reference books list them as being given with 'special precautions' during pregnancy, while the American Physicians' Desk Reference state that they should not be used in pregnancy. However, as many as 35 per cent of pregnant women can be given these tranquillisers for insomnia and anxiety problems.[257] Babies born from mothers who have taken these drugs have problems such as dyslexia and attention deficit hyperactive disorder.[258]

In conclusion, I think we should learn from the thalidomide disaster that drugs can be extremely potent, especially when taken at the most crucial times of cell division (normally in the early part of pregnancy).

However, it is important to realise that it is possible to prevent foetal damage due to most of the causes discussed in this section of the book. Now that you are armed with accurate information, you can take action to protect yourself and your child throughout your pregnancy and later on.

CHAPTER 25

Looking Forward to Becoming a Parent

It has become clearer from recent research that a number of problems experienced during pregnancy or even in the baby's health could be prevented. If you do the best you can with your nutrition and lifestyle, environment, etc you are giving your baby the best possible chance of being healthy.

Taking the time to make changes before conception and carrying them through pregnancy may seem at times like a lot of effort. But science is now showing us that that effort is well rewarded not in just getting pregnant in the first place but keeping you and your baby healthy through pregnancy. It is also now recognised that the environment in the womb has an enormous impact on the future health of the baby and possibly intellectual development. It is a small price to pay for you and your partner to get yourselves into optimum health before conception to create a healthy human being.

Glossary

amino acid – Building blocks of the body which are different forms of protein

androgens – Hormones that increase male characteristics e.g. testosterone

anovulation – Failure of the ovaries to produce, mature or release eggs

antioxidants – Compounds that stop oxidation when a substance is exposed to oxygen which can create highly reactive chemical fragments called free radicals. These free radicals have been linked to cancer, coronary heart disease and premature ageing.

basal body temperature – Temperature taken when the body is at rest

Body Mass Index – A ratio of height to weight: weight in kg divided by the square of your height in metres

chromosome – A strand of DNA that carries the genes determining hereditary

clomiphene – An anti-oestrogen drug used to induce ovulation

coeliac disease – A condition caused by an intolerance to gluten which prevents food being absorbed properly. Symptoms can include foul-smelling greasy stools, weight loss, anaemia, bloating, fatigue and signs of multiple vitamin and minerals deficiencies.

complex carbohydrates – Carbohydrates are organic compounds which are the main source of energy for the body. The more complex they are the more 'slow burning' and so they give a sustainable level of energy. Examples are wholemeal bread, brown rice, pasta oats and vegetables.

corpus luteum – A structure that grows with the follicle after the egg has been released at ovulation. It secretes progesterone which helps to maintain pregnancy.

donor eggs – Eggs which are donated by another woman, usually anonymously, to be used in IVF or ICSI treatment when a woman cannot produce her own eggs or the quality is poor

donor sperm – Sperm donated by a man usually anonymously to be used in assisted conception

embryo – The name usually used for a developing human up to the seventh or eighth week of pregnancy

endometriosis – A medical condition that causes the lining of the womb to grow elsewhere in the body

essential fatty acids (essential fats) – Unsaturated fats that are essential for health. They are found in nuts, seeds, oily fish and vegetables.

fallopian tubes – The tubes which capture the egg as it is released from the ovary, and where fertilisation takes place

fertilisation – The union of the egg and the sperm to form an embryo

foetus – The word used for a developing human being after approximately the eighth week of pregnancy

fibroids – Benign tumours which grow in the womb

foetal alcohol syndrome – A condition in the baby caused by the mother consuming alcohol during pregnancy. It is characterised by certain physical abnormalities and retarded development.

follicle stimulating hormone (FSH) – The hormone secreted from the pituitary gland in the brain which begins the process of ovulation by stimulating the ovaries to produce oestrogen

genetically modified (GM) foods – Foods where genes from another species are introduced into a particular plant to make them more resistant to pests, viruses or weed killers. In order to smuggle these new genes across the species barrier, scientists use infectious agents (viruses and bacteria). Then antibiotic resistant genes are used as genetic markers to allow the scientists to track the movements of these new genes once inserted.

genito-urinary infections – Infections related to the genital (reproductive) and urinary (bladder etc) systems of the body

GIFT (Gamete Intra Fallopian Transfer) – An assisted conception technique, where the egg and sperm are mixed together (not fertilised) and then put back into the fallopian tubes so that fertilisation takes place where it would happen naturally anyway.

HFEA (Human Fertilisation and Embryo Authority) – licenses clinics to do assisted conception techniques such as IVF

ICSI (Intracytoplasmic Sperm Injection) – This is when a single sperm is injected directly into the egg to fertilise it. The embryo is then implanted in the womb.

IUI (Intrauterine Insemination) – A procedure that puts your partners sperm directly into your womb at a much higher level than can be achieved during intercourse to improve the chances of fertilisation

IVF (In-vitro Fertilisation) – A technique for fertilising your eggs with your partner's sperm outside your body. The fertilised egg is then implanted back into your womb.

luteinising hormone (LH) – The hormone released by the pituitary gland which triggers ovulation

oestrogen – A group of hormones that is responsible for the development of female characteristics such as breast development and during each menstrual cycle thickens the lining of the womb.

ovulation – The release of an egg (ovum) from the ovary.

phyto-oestrogens – Plant hormones that exert weak oestrogenic activity

polycystic ovary syndrome – A condition where the ovaries are larger than normal and the undeveloped follicles resemble a bunch of grapes. There is an accompanying hormone imbalance which results in symptoms such as weight gain, body hair, skin problems and mood swings.

progesterone – The hormone that is released by the corpus luteum during the second half of the cycle which helps to maintain a pregnancy once fertilisation has taken place

prostaglandins – Hormone-like regulating substances which play a part in inflammatory responses in the body

sperm count – The number of sperm per millilitre which should be more than 20 million

testosterone – The hormone responsible for the development of male characteristics

trans fats – Fats that are produced from the process of hydrogenation in food manufacturing

ultrasound – The use of very high frequency sound waves to obtain images of structures within the body

varicoceles – Varicose veins within the testes which may affect sperm production

xenoestrogens – Foreign oestrogens which are produced from the plastic and pesticide industries

References

1 Carlsen, E. et al, 'Evidence for decreasing quality of semen during the past 50 years', *British Medical Journal*, vol 305 (1992), pp. 609–13.

2 The MRC Vitamin Study Group, 'Prevention of neural tube defects – Results of the Medical Research Council Vitamin Study', *Lancet*, vol 238 (1991), pp. 131–7.

3 Nelson, M.M. and Evans, H.M., 'Pteroylglutamic acid and reproduction in the rat', *Journal of Nutrition*, vol 38 (1949), pp. 11–24.
Giroud, A. and Lefebvres-Boisselot, J., 'Anomalies provoqués chez le foetus en l'absence d'acide folique', *Archives Francaises de Pediatrie*, vol 8 (1951), pp. 648–56.

4 Lawrence, K.N. et al, 'Double-blind randomised controlled trial of folate treatment before conception to prevent recurrence of neural tube defects', *British Medical Journal*, vol 282 (1981), pp. 1509–51.

5 *Daily Mail* (23 November 1993).

6 'Preconceptual care and pregnancy outcome', *Journal of Nutritional and Environmental Medicine*, vol 5 (1995), pp. 205–8.

7 Schroeder, H.A., 'Losses of vitamins and trace minerals, resulting from processing and preservation of foods', *American Journal of Clinical Nutrition*, vol 24 (1971), pp. 562–73.

8 Frisch, R.E., 'What's below the surface?', *New England Journal of Medicine*, vol 305 (1981), pp. 1019–20.

9 Vigersky, B.A. et al, 'Hypothalamic dysfunction in secondary amenorrhea associated with simple weight loss', *New England Journal of Medicine*, vol 297 (1977), pp. 1141–5.

10 Foreyt, J.P. and Poston, W.S., 'Obesity: a never-ending cycle?', *International Journal of Fertility and Women's Medicine*, vol 43(2) (1998), pp. 111–16.

11 Clark, A.M. et al, 'Weight loss results in significant improvement in pregnancy and ovulation rates in anovulatory obese women', *Human Reproduction*, vol 10 (1995), pp. 2705–12.

12 Bennet, H.S. et al, 'Breast and prostate in men who die of cirrhosis of the liver', *American Journal of Clinical Pathology*, vol 20 (1950), pp. 814–28.

13 Mendelson, J.M., 'Effects of alcohol on plasma testosterone and luteinising hormone levels', *Alcoholism Clinical & Experimental Research*, vol 2 (1978), pp. 225–58.

14 Abbasi, A.A. et al, 'Experimental zinc deficiency in man: effect on testicular function', *Journal of Laboratory and Clinical Medicine*, vol 96(3) (1980), pp. 544–50.

15 Hughes, J.M. et al, 'Hypothalamo-pituitary ovarian function in thirty-one women with chronic alcoholism', *Clinical Endocrinology (Oxford)*, vol 12 (1980), pp. 543–51.

Valimake, M. et al, 'Sex hormones in amenorrheic women with alcoholic liver disease', *Journal of Clinical Endocrinology and Metabolism*, vol 59 (1984), pp. 133–8.

16 Jensen, T. et al, 'Does moderate alcohol consumption affect fertility? Follow-up study among couples planning first pregnancy', *British Medical Journal*, vol 317 (1998), pp. 505–10.

17 Hakim, R. et al, 'Alcohol and caffeine consumption and decreased fertility', *Fertility and Sterility*, vol 70(4) (1998), pp. 632–7.

18 Kline, J. et al, 'Smoking: A risk factor for spontaneous abortion', *New England Journal of Medicine*, vol 297 (1977), pp. 793–6.

19 Gonzales, E., 'Sperm swim singly after vitamin C therapy' *Journal of the American Medical Association*, vol 249 (1983), p. 2747.

20 Campbell, J.M. and Harrison, 'Smoking and Infertility', *Medical Journal of Australia*, vol 1 (1979), pp. 342–3.

21 Jick, H. et al, 'Relation between smoking and age of natural menopause', *Lancet*, vol 1 (1977), pp. 1354–5.

22 Powell, D.J. and Fuller, R.W., 'Marijuana and sex: strange bed partners', *Journal of Psychoactive Drugs*, vol 15 (1983), pp. 169–280.

23 Ibid.

24 Bracken, M.B. et al, 'Association of cocaine use with sperm concentration, motility and morphology', *Fertility and Sterility*, vol 53 (1990), pp. 315–22.

25 Smith, C.G. and Gilbean, P.M., 'Drug abuse effects on reproductive hormones' in J. Thomas et al (eds), *Endocrine Toxicology*, Raven Press, New York (1985).

26 Bongol, N. et al, 'Teratogenicity of cocaine in humans', *Journal of Pediatrics*, vol 1 (1987), pp. 93–6.
Ostrea, E.M. and Chavez, C.J. 'Perinatal problems (excluding neonatal withdrawal) in maternal drug addiction: a study of 830 cases', *Journal of Pediatrics*, vol 94 (1979), pp. 292–5.

27 *The Initial Investigation and Management of the Infertile Couple: Evidence-Based Clinical Guidelines No 2*, Royal College of Obstetricians and Gynaecologists (February 1998).

28 Ibid.

29 Hull, M.G.R., 'Epidemiology of infertility and polycystic ovarian disease: endocrinological and demographic studies', *Gynaecological Endocrinology*, vol 1 (1987), pp. 235–45.

30 Sher, K.S. and Mayberry, J.F., *Acta Paediatrica. Supplement*, vol 412 (1996), pp. 76–7.

31 Ahlgren, M. et al, 'Sperm transport and survival in women with special reference to the Fallopian tube, The Biology of Spermatazoa', INSERM International Symposium, Nouzilly, Karger, Basel (1975), pp. 63–73.

32 Jones, G.E.S. and Delfs, E., 'Endocrine patterns in term pregnancies following abortion', *Journal of the American Medical Association*, vol 146 (1951), pp. 1212–18.

33 Bonde, J.P. et al, 'Relation between semen quality and fertility: a population based study', *Lancet*, vol 352 (1998), pp. 1172–7.

34 Alder, M.W., *ABC of sexually transmitted diseases*, British Medical Association, London (1984).

35 Royal College of Physicians Committee on Genito-urinary Medicine, 'Chlamydial diagnostic services in the UK and Eire: current facilities and perceived needs', *Genitourinary Medicine*, vol 62 (1987), pp. 371–4.

36 Berger, R.E. et al, 'Chlamydia trachomatis as a cause of "idiopathic" epididymitis', *New England Journal of Medicine*, vol 298 (1978), pp. 301–4.

37 Suominen, J. et al, 'Chronic prostatitis, chlamydia trachomatis and infertility', *International Journal of Andrology*, vol 6 (1983), pp. 405–13.

38 Gnarpe, H. and Friberg, J., 'Mycoplasma and human reproductive failure', *American Journal of Obstetric Gynecology*, vol 114 (1972), p. 727.

39 Gnarpe, H. and Friberg, J., 'Mycoplasma infections and infertility' in R.E. Mancini and L. Martini (eds), *Male Fertility and Sterility*, vol 5 (1974).

40 Fowlkes, D.M. et al, 'T-mycoplasmas and human infertility: correlation of infection with alternations in seminal parameters', *Fertility and Sterility*, vol 26 (1975), p. 1212.
Bercovici, B. et al, 'Isolation of mycoplasmas from the genital tract of women with reproductive failure', *Israel Journal of Medical Sciences*, vol 14 (1978), p. 347.
Stray-Pedersen, B. et al, 'Uterine mycoplasma colonisation in reproductive failure', *American Journal of Obstetrics and Gynecology*, vol 130 (1978), p. 307.

41 Quinn, P.A. et al, 'Serologic evidence of ureaplasma urealyticum infection in women with spontaneous pregnancy loss', *American Journal of Obstetrics and Gynecology*, vol 145 (1983), pp. 245–50.

42 Gerhard, I. et al, 'Prolonged exposure to wood preservative induces endocrine and immunologic disorders in women', *American Journal of Obstetrics and Gynecology*, vol 165(2) (1991), pp. 487–8.

43 Rowley, M.J. et al, 'Effects of graded doses of ionising irradiation on the human testis', *Radiation Research*, vol 59 (1974), p. 665.

44 Sandeman, T.F. 'The effects of X-irradiation on male human fertility', *British Journal of Radiology*, vol 39 (1966), p. 901.

45 Oldereid, N.G. et al, 'Male infertility. Significance of life and occupation', *Tidsskrift for Den Norske Laegeforening*, vol 114 (1994), pp. 3308–11.

46 Youbicier-Smio, B.J. et al, 'Biological effects of continuous exposure of embryos and young chickens to electromagnetic fields emitted by video display units', *Bioelectromagnetics*, vol 18(7) (1997), pp. 514–23.

47 *Green Farm Magazine* (Winter 1990).

48 Schrumpf, F. and Charley, H., 'Texture of broccoli and carrots cooked by microwave energy', *Journal of Food Science*, vol 40 (1975), pp. 1025–9.

49 Rowland, A.S. et al, 'The effect of occupational exposure to mercury vapour on the fertility of female dental assistants', *Occupational and Environmental Medicine*, vol 51(1) (1994), pp. 28–34.

50 *Green Farm Magazine* (Winter 1990).

51 Dickman, M.D. and Leung, K.M., 'Mercury and organochlorine exposure from fish consumption in Hong Kong', *Chemosphere*, vol 37(5) (1998), pp. 991–1015.

52 Bryce-Smith, D. and Waldron, H.A., 'Lead pollution, disease and behaviour', *Community Health*, vol 6 (1974), pp. 168–75.

53 Winder, C., 'Lead, reproduction and development', *Neurotoxicology*, vol 14 (1993), p. 303.

54 Tabacova, S. and Balabaeva, L., *Environmental Health Perspectives Supplements*, vol 101(2) (1993), pp. 27–31.

55 Coste, J. et al, 'Lead-exposed workmen and fertility: a cohort study on 354 subjects', *European Journal of Epidemiology*, vol 7 (1991), pp. 154–8.

56 Sas, M. and Szollosi, J., 'Impaired spermatogenesis as a common finding among professional drivers', *Archives of Andrology*, vol 3 (1979), p. 57.

57 Bonde, J.P., 'The risk of male subfertility attributable to welding of metals – studies of semen quality, infertility, fertility, adverse pregnancy outcome and childhood malignancy', *International Journal of Andrology*, vol 16 (1993), p. 1.

58 Henderson, J. et al, 'Association between occupational group and sperm concentration in infertile men', *Clinical Reproduction and Fertility*, vol 4 (1986), p. 275.

Hemminki, K. et al, 'Spontaneous abortion by occupation and social class in Finland', *International Journal of Epidemiology*, vol 9 (1980), p. 149.

59 Thrupp, L.A., 'Sterilisation of workers from pesticide exposure: the causes and consequences of DBCP-induced damage in Costa Rica and beyond', *International Journal of the Health Sciences*, vol 21(4) (1991), pp. 731–57.

60 Olsen, G.W. et al, 'Determinants of spermatogenesis recovery among workers exposed to 1,2-dibromo-3-chloropropane', *Journal of Occupational Medicine*, vol 32 (1990), pp. 979–84.

61 Gerhard, I. et al, 'Toxic pollutants and fertility disorders: solvents and pesticides', *Geburtshilfe – Frauenheilkd*, vol 53(3) (1993), pp. 147–60.

62 Baranski, B., *Environmental Health Perspectives Supplements*, vol 101(2) (1993), pp. 81–90.

63 Paul, M., 'Occupational Reproductive Hazards', *Lancet*, vol 349 (1997), pp. 1385–8.

64 Goldhaber, M.K. et al, 'The risk of miscarriage and birth defects among women who use visual display terminals during pregnancy', *American Journal of Industrial Medicine*, vol 13 (1988), pp. 695–706.

65 Brix, K. et al, 'Study of 4215 clerical employees in Michigan', presented at APHA meeting, University of Michigan (1986).

66 'Japanese miscarriages blamed on computer terminals' *New Scientist* (23 May 1985).

67 Giblin, P.T. et al, 'Effects of stress and characteristic adaptability on semen quality in healthy men', *Fertility and Sterility*, vol 49 (1988), pp. 127–32.

68 Negro-Vilar, A., *Environmental Health Perspectives Supplements*, vol 101(2) (1993), pp. 59–64.

69 Barnea, E.R. and Tal, J., 'Stress-related reproductive failure', *Journal of In Vitro Fertilisation and Embryo Transfer*, vol 8 (1991), pp. 15–23.

70 Menninger, K., 'Somatic correlations with the unconscious repudiation of femininity in women', *Journal of Nervous and Mental Disease*, vol 89 (1939), p. 514.
Benedeck, T. and Rubenstein, B., 'Correlations between ovarian activity and psychodynamic processes. The anovulatory phase', *Psychosomatic Medicine*, vol 1(2) (1939), pp. 245–70.

71 Perloff, W.H. and Steinberger, E., 'In vivo survival of spermatazoa in cervical mucus', *American Journal of Obstetrics and Gynecology*, vol 88 (1964), pp. 439–42.

72 Ziegler, J., 'Soybeans show promise in cancer prevention', *Journal of the National Cancer Institute*, vol 86 (1994), pp. 1666–7.

73 Cassidy, A. et al, 'Biological effects of a diet of soy protein rich in isoflavones on the menstrual cycle of premenopausal women', *American Journal of Clinical Nutrition*, vol 60 (1994), pp. 333–40.

74 Wilcox, A. et al, 'Caffeinated beverages and decreased fertility', *Lancet*, vol 2 (1988), pp. 1453–5.

75 Stanton, C. and Gray, R., 'Effects of caffeine consumption on delayed conception', *American Journal of Epidemiology*, vol 142(12) (1995), pp. 1322–9.
Hatch, E.E. and Bracken, M.B., 'Association of delayed conception with caffeine consumption', *American Journal of Epidemiology*, vol 138 (1993), pp. 1082–92.
Boulmar, F. et al, 'Caffeine intake and delayed conception: A European multicentre study on infertility and subfecundity, European Study Group on Infertility and Subfecundity', *American Journal of Epidemiology*, vol 145(4) (1997), pp. 324–34.

76 Parazzini, F. et al, 'Risk factors for unexplained dyspermia in infertile men: a case-control study', *Archives of Andrology*, vol 31(2) (1993), pp. 105–13.

77 Ingram, D.J., *Journal of the National Cancer Institute*, vol 79 (1987), p. 1225.

78 *Lancet* (21 May 1994).

79 Srivastava, K.C. et al, 'Prostaglandin E and 19-hydroxy-prostaglandin E content in the semen of men with normal sperm characteristics, men with abnormal sperm characteristics, vasectomised men and polyzoospermic men', *Danish Medical Bulletin*, vol 28 (1981), pp. 201–3.

80 Vander Walt, L.A. et al, 'Unusual sex hormone pattern among desert-dwelling hunter-gatherers', *Journal of Clinical Endocrinology and Metabolism*, vol 46 (1978), p. 658.

81 Pirke, K.M. et al, 'The influence of dieting on the menstrual cycle of healthy young women', *Journal of Clinical Endocrinology and Metabolism*, vol 60 (1985), pp. 1174–9.

82 Bates, G.W. et al, 'Reproductive failure in women who practise weight control', *Fertility and Sterility*, vol 37(3) (1982), pp. 373–8.

83 *American Journal of Clinical Nutrition*, vol 64 (1996), p. 4.

84 Wynn, A. and Wynn, M., 'The need for nutritional assessment in the treatment of the infertile patient', *Journal of Nutritional Medicine*, vol 1 (1990), pp. 315–24.

85 Foreyt, J.P. and Poston, W.S., 'Obesity: a never-ending cycle?' *International Journal of Fertility and Women's Medicine*, vol 43(2) (1998), pp. 111–16.

86 Clarm, A.M. et al, 'Weight loss results in significant improvement in pregnancy and ovulation rates in anovulatory obese women', *Human Reproduction*, vol 10(1) (1995), pp. 2705–12.

87 Kiddy, D.S. et al, 'Diet-induced changes in sex hormone binding globulin and free testosterone in women with normal or polycystic ovaries: correlation with serum insulin and insulin-like growth factor-I', *Clinical Endocrinology*, vol 31 (1989), pp. 757–63.

88 Van Thiel, D.M., 'Hypogonadism in alcoholic liver disease: Evidence for a double effect', *Gastroenterology*, vol 67 (1974), pp. 1188–99.

89 Wynn, M. and Wynn, A., *The Case for Preconception Care for Men and Women*, AB Academic Publishers (1991).

90 Ward, N. et al, 'Placental element levels in relation to foetal development of obstetrically normal births: A study of 37 elements. Evidence for effects of cadmium, lead and zinc on foetal growth, and smoking as a cause of cadmium', *International Journal of Biosocial Research*, vol 9(1) (1987), p. 63081.

91 Sorahan, T. et al, 'Childhood cancer and parental use of tobacco: deaths from 1971 to 1976', *British Journal of Cancer*, vol 76(11) (1997), pp. 1525–31.

92 Murray, M. and Pizzorno, J., *Encyclopaedia of Natural Medicine*, Prima (1991).

93 Wald, N.J. and Bower, C., 'Folic acid, pernicious anaemia and neural tube defects', *Lancet*, vol 343 (1994), p. 307.

94 Shaw, F.M. et al, 'Risks of orofacial clefts in children born to women using multivitamins containing folic acid preconceptually', *Lancet*, vol 346 (1995), pp. 393–6.

95 Russel, R.M., 'A minimum of 13,500 deaths annually from coronary artery disease could be prevented by increasing folate intake in order to reduce homocysteine levels', *Journal of the American Medical Association*, vol 275 (1996), pp. 1828–9.

96 Krause, M.V. and Mahan, K.L., *Food, Nutrition and Diet Therapy*, seventh edition, W.B. Saunders, Philadelphia (1984).

97 Schwabe, J.W.R. and Rhodes, D., 'Beyond zinc fingers: steroid hormone receptors have a novel structure motif for DNA recognition', *Trends in Biochemical Science*, vol 16 (1991), pp. 291–6.

98 Hurley, L.S., 'Teratogenic aspects of manganese, zinc and copper nutrition', *Physiological Reviews*, vol 61 (1991), pp. 249–95.

99 Taumara, T. et al, 'Absorption of mono and polyglutamyl folates in zinc-depleted men', *American Journal of Clinical Nutrition*, vol 31 (1978), p. 1984.

100 Davies, S., 'Zinc, nutrition and health', in E. Bland (ed), *1984–1985 Yearbook of Nutritional Medicine*, Keats Publishing, New Canaan, Connecticut (1985), pp. 113–52.

101 Dinsale, D. and Williams, R.B., 'Ultrastructural changes in the sperm tail of zinc-deficient rats', *Journal of Comparative Pathology*, vol 90 (1980), pp. 559–66.

102 Taneja, S.K. and Nirmal, A., 'Histopathology of testes of mice fed on zinc-deficient diet', *Indian Journal of Experimental Biology*, vol 18 (1980), pp. 1411–14.

103 Abbasi, A.A. et al, 'Experimental zinc deficiency in man: effect on testicular function', *Journal of Laboratory and Clinical Medicine*, vol 96 (1980), pp. 544–50.
Piesse, J., 'Zinc and human male infertility', *International Clinical Nutrition Review*, vol 3 (1983), pp. 4–6.

104 Hunt, C.D. et al, 'Effects of dietary zinc depletion on seminal volume and zinc loss, serum testosterone concentration, and sperm morphology in young men', *American Journal of Clinical Nutrition*, vol 56 (1992), pp. 148–57.

105 Netter, A. et al, 'Effect of zinc administration on plasma testosterone, dihydrotestosterone and sperm count', *Archives of Andrology*, vol 7 (1981), pp. 69–73.

106 Mohan, H. et al, 'Inter-relationship of zinc levels in serum and semen in oligospermic infertile patients and fertile males', *Indian Journal of Pathology and Microbiology*, vol 40(4) (1997), pp. 451–5.

107 Hunt, C.D. et al, 'Effects of dietary zinc depletion on seminal volume and zinc loss, serum testosterone concentration and sperm morphology in young men', *American Journal of Clinical Nutrition*, vol 56(1) (1992), pp. 148–57.

108 Scott, R. et al, 'Selenium supplementation in subfertile human males', in P.W.F. Fischer et al (eds), *Trace Elements in man and animals – 9 (TEMA 9)*, Ottawa NRC Research Press (1997).

109 Krznjavi, H. et al, 'Selenium and fertility in men', *Trace Elements in Medicine*, vol 9(2) (1992), pp. 107–8.

110 Srivastava, K.C. et al, 'Prostaglandin E and 19-hydroxy-prostaglandin E content in the semen of men with normal sperm characteristics, men with abnormal sperm characteristics, vasectomised men and polyzoospermic men', *Danish Medical Bulletin*, vol 28 (1981), pp. 201–3.

111 Rossi, E. and Costa, M., 'Fish oil derivatives as a prophylaxis of recurrent miscarriages associated with antiphospholipid antibodies: a pilot study', *Lupus*, vol 2(5) (1993), pp. 319–23.

112 Rice, R., 'Fish and healthy pregnancy: more than just a red herring', *Professional Care of Mother and Baby*, vol 6(6) (1996), pp. 171–3.

113 Reece, M.S. et al, 'Maternal and Perinatal Long-Chain Fatty Acids: Possible roles in preterm birth', *American Journal of Obstetrics and Gynecology*, vol 176(4) (1997), pp. 907–14.

114 Kidd, G.S. et al, 'The effects of pyridoxine on pituitary hormone secretion in amenorrhea-galactorrhea syndromes', *Journal of Clinical Endocrinology and Metabolism*, vol 54(4) (1982), pp. 872–5.

115 Abraham, G.E. and Hargrove, J.T., reported in *Medical World News* (19 March 1979).

116 Kumamoto, Y. et al, 'Clinical efficacy of mecobalamin in treatment of oligospermia. Results of a double-blind comparative clinical study', *Alta Urological Japonica*, vol 34 (1988), pp. 1109–32.

117 Sandler, B. and Faragher, B., 'Treatment of oligospermia with vitamin B12', *Infertility*, vol 7 (1984), pp. 133–8.

118 Geva, E. et al, 'The effect of anti-oxidant treatment on human spermatozoa and fertilisa-

tion rate in an in vitro fertilisation program', *Fertility and Sterility*, vol 66(3) (1996), pp. 430–4.

119 Aitken, R.J. et al, 'Analysis of the relationship between defective sperm function and the generation of reactive oxygen species in cases of oligozoospermia', *Journal of Andrology*, vol 10 (1989), pp. 214–20.

120 Bayer, R., 'Treatment of infertility with vitamin E', *International Journal of Infertility*, vol 5 (1960), pp. 70–8.

121 Tarin, J. et al, 'Effects of maternal ageing and dietary anti-oxidant supplementation on ovulation, fertilisation and embryo development in vitro in the mouse', *Reproduction, Nutrition, Development*, vol 38(5) (1998), pp. 499–508.

122 Fraga, C.G. et al, 'Ascorbic acid protects against endogenous oxidative DNA damage in human sperm', *Proceedings of the National Academy of Science*, vol 88 (1991), pp. 11003–6.

123 'Daily vitamin C protects sperm from genetic damage', *Medical Tribune* (16 and 23 January 1992).

124 Gonzales, E.R., 'Sperm swim singly after vitamin C therapy', *Journal of the American Medical Association*, vol 20 (1983), p. 2727.
Dawson, E.B. et al, 'Effect of ascorbic acid on sperm fertility', *Federal Proceedings*, vol 42, abstract # 31403 (1983), p. 531.

125 Dawson, E.B. et al, 'Effect of ascorbic acid on male fertility', *Annals of New York Academy of Science*, vol 498 (1987), pp. 812–28.

126 Igarashi, I., 'Augmentative effects of ascorbic acid upon induction of human ovulation in clomiphene ineffective anovulatory women', *International Journal of Fertility*, vol 22(3) (1977), pp. 68–73.

127 Podmore, I. et al, 'Vitamin C exhibits pro-oxidant effect', *Nature*, vol 392 (1998), p. 559.

128 Levine, M. et al, 'Does vitamin C have a pro-oxidant effect?' *Nature*, vol 395 (1998), p. 231.

129 Saner, G. et al, 'Hair manganese concentrations in newborns and their mothers', *American Journal of Clinical Nutrition*, vol 41 (1985), pp. 1042–4.

130 Rushton, D.H. et al, letter to *Ferritin and fertility*, *Lancet*, vol 337 (1991), p. 1554.

131 *Miscarriage Association Newsletter* (1992).

132 Taymore, M.L. et al, 'The aetiological role of chronic iron deficiency in production of menorrhagia', *Journal of the American Medical Association*, vol 187 (1964), pp. 323–7.

133 Sullivan, J.L, 'Stored iron and ischemic heart disease', editorial in *Circulation*, vol 86 (1992), p. 1036.

134 Borigato, E.V. and Martinez, F.E., 'Iron nutritional status is improved in Brazilian preterm infants fed food cooked in iron pots', *Journal of Nutrition*, vol 128(5) (1998), pp. 855–9.

135 Park, J. and Brittin, H.C., 'Increased iron content of food due to stainless cookware', *Journal of the American Dietetic Association*, vol 97(6) (1997), pp. 659–61.

136 Holt Jr, L.E. and Albanese, A.A. 'Observations on amino acid deficiencies in man', *Transactions of the Association of American Physicians*, vol 58 (1944), p. 143.

137 Bridge, C., 'The Administration of L-arginine to enhance male fertility', dissertation for the Institute of Optimum Nutrition Diploma Course (1998).

138 de Aloysio, D. et al, 'The clinical use of arginine aspartate in male infertility', *Alta Europaea Fertilitatis*, vol 13 (1982), pp. 133–67.
Tanimura, J. 'Studies on arginine in human semen. Part II. The effects of medication with L-arginine-HCl on male infertility', *Bulletin of Osaka Medical School*, vol 13 (1967), pp. 84–9.

139 Schater, A. et al, 'Treatment of ligospermia with the amino acid arginine', *Journal of Urology*, vol 110 (1973), pp. 311–13.

140 Gaby, A.R., *Townsend Letters for Doctors and Patients* (April 1996), p. 20.

141 Costa, M. et al, 'L-carnitine in idiopathic asthenozoospermia: A multicentre study', *Andrologia*, vol 26 (1994), pp. 155–9.

142 Vitali, G. et al, 'Carnitine supplementation in human idiopathic asthenospermia. Clinical Results', *Drugs Under Experimental and Clinical Research*, vol 21 (1995), pp. 157–9.

143 Rothman et al, *New England Journal of Medicine*, vol 333(21) (1995), pp. 157–9.

144 Jennings, I., *Vitamins in Endocrine Metabolism*, Heinemann (1972).

145 West, K.P. et al, 'Double-blind, cluster randomised trial of low dose supplementation with vitamin A or beta-carotene on mortality related to pregnancy in Nepal', *British Medical Journal*, vol 318 (1999), pp. 570–5.

146 Sliutz, G. et al, 'Agnus castus extracts inhibit prolactin secretion of rat pituitary cells', *Hormone and Metabolic Research*, vol 25 (1993), pp. 253–5.

147 Propping, D. and Katzorke, T., 'Treatment of corpus luteum insufficiency', *Zeitschr Allgemeinmedizin*, vol 63 (1987), pp. 932–3.

148 Handley, R., *Homeopathy for Women*, Thorsons (1993).

149 Suzuki, T. and Yamamoto, P., 'Organic mercury levels in human hair with and without storage for eleven years', *Bulletin of Environmental Contamination and Toxicology*, vol 28 (1982), pp. 186–8.

150 Dickman, M.D. and Leung, K.M., 'Mercury and organochlorine exposure from fish consumption in Hong Kong', *Chemosphere*, vol 37(5) (1998), pp. 991–1015.

151 Vallee, B., 'Zinc' in C.L. Comar and C.S. Bonner (eds), *Mineral metabolism*, vol IIB, Academic Press (1965).

152 Sonnenbichler, J. and Zetl, I., 'Stimulating influence of a flavonolignan derivative on proliferation, RNA synthesis and protein synthesis in liver cells', in L. Okolicsanyi, G. Cosmos and G. Crepaldi (eds), *Assessment and Management of Hepatobiliary Disease*, Springer-Verlag, Berlin (1987), pp. 263–72.

153 Boyce, N., 'Growing up too soon', *New Scientist* (2 August 1997), p. 5.

154 Chivers, C. et al, 'Apparent doubling of frequency of undescended testes in England and Wales in 1962–1981', *Lancet*, vol ii (1984), pp. 330–2.

155 Giwercman, A. and Skakkebaek, N.E., 'The human testes: An organ at risk?', *International Journal of Andrology*, vol 15 (1992), pp. 373–5.

156 Abell, A. et al, 'High sperm density among members of organic farmers' association', *Lancet*, vol 343(8911) (1994), p. 1498.

157 Bryce-Smith, D., 'Lead-induced disorders and mentation in children', *Nutrition and Health*, vol 1 (1983), pp. 179–94.

158 Robinson, D. and Rock, J., 'Intrascrotal hyperthermia induced by isolation effect on spermatogenesis', *Obstetrics and Gynaecology*, vol 29 (1967), p. 217.

159 *Lancet* (20 January 1996).

160 Werbach, M., *Nutritional Influences on Illness*, Third Line Press (1996).

161 Regan, L., *Miscarriage*, Bloomsbury Publishing (1997).

162 Ibid.

163 Kiddy, D.S. et al, 'Differences in clinical and endocrine features between obese and non-obese subjects with polycystic ovary syndrome: an analysis of 263 consecutive cases', *Clinical Endocrinology*, vol 32 (1990), pp. 213–20.

164 Kiddy, D.S. et al, 'Diet-induced changes in sex hormone binding globulin and free testosterone in women with normal or polycystic ovaries; correlation with serum insulin and insulin-like growth factor-I', *Clinical Endocrinology*, vol 31 (1989), pp. 757–63.

165 Kiddy, D.S. et al, 'Improvement in endocrine and ovarian function during dietary treat-

ment of obese women with polycystic ovary syndrome', *Clinical Endocrinology*, vol 36 (1992), pp. 105–11.

166 Clark, A.M. et al, 'Weight loss results in significant improvement in pregnancy and ovulation rates in anovulatory obese women', *Human Reproduction*, vol 10 (1995), pp. 2705–12.

167 Ingram, D.J., *Journal of the National Cancer Institute*, vol 79 (1987), p. 1225.

168 Grodstein, F. et al, 'Relation of female infertility to consumption of caffeinated beverages', *American Journal of Epidemiology*, vol 137 (1993), pp. 1353–60.

169 Bernstein, L., *Journal of the National Cancer Institute*, vol 137 (1994), p. 18.

170 Wagner, H., in J.L. Beal and E. Reinhard (eds), *Natural Products as Medicinal Agents* (1981).

171 Mathias, J.R. et al, 'Relation of endometriosis and neuromuscular disease of the gastrointestinal tract: new insights', *Fertility and Sterility*, vol 70 (1998), pp. 81–7.

172 Furuhjelm et al, 'The quality of human semen in spontaneous abortion', *International Journal of Fertility*, vol 7 (1962), pp. 17–21.

173 Guid Oei, S. et al, 'Effectiveness of the post-coital test: randomised controlled trial', *British Medical Journal*, vol 317 (1998), pp. 502–5.

174 Alder, M.W., *ABC of sexually transmitted diseases*, British Medical Association (1984).

175 Blattner, R.J., 'The role of viruses in congenital defects', *American Journal of Diseases of Childhood*, vol 128 (1974), pp. 781–6.

176 Ho-Yen, D.O., 'Toxoplasma and cytomegalovirus infections during pregnancy', *Maternal and Child Health* (August 1988), pp. 225–7.

177 Weidner, W., 'Ureaplasmal infections of the male urogenital tract, in particular prostatitis and semen quality', *Urology International*, vol 40 (1982), pp. 42–5.

178 Swenson, C.E. et al, 'Ureaplasma urealyticum and human fertility: the effect of antibiotic therapy on semen quality', *Fertility and Sterility*, vol 31 (1979), pp. 660–5.

179 Sutton, G., 'Genital infection', *Midwife, Health Visitor and Community Nurse*, 18(2) (1982), pp. 42–5.

180 Multidisciplinary Working Group, *Prenatal screening for toxoplasmosis in the UK*, Royal College of Obstetricians and Gynaecologists (1992).

181 Gibbs, R.S., 'Microbiology of the female genital tract', *American Journal of Obstetrics and Gynecology*, vol 156 (1987), pp. 491–5.

182 Villar, J. et al, 'Nutritional and antimicrobial interventions to prevent preterm birth: an overview of randomised controlled trials', *Obstetrical and Gynaecological Survey*, vol 53(9) (1998), pp. 575–85.

183 Morton, R.F., 'Candidal vaginitis: Natural history, predisposing factors and prevention', *Proceedings of the Royal Society of Medicine*, vol 70(4) (1977), pp. 3–6.

184 Fratta, I.D. et al, 'Teratogenic effect of thalidomide in rabbits, rats, hamsters and mice', *Toxicology and Applied Pharmacology*, vol 7 (1965), pp. 268–86.

185 Jackson, A.J. and Schumacher, H.J., 'The teratogenic activity of a thalidomide analogus EM12 in rats on a low zinc diet', *Teratology*, vol 19 (1979), pp. 341–4.

186 Rossing, M.A. et al, 'Ovarian tumours in a cohort of infertile women', *New England Journal of Medicine*, vol 331 (1994), pp. 771–6.

187 *The Management of Infertility in Secondary Care, Evidence Based Clinical Guidelines No. 3*, The Royal College of Obstetricians and Gynaecologists (1998).

188 Ibid.

189 Bals-Pratsch, M. et al, 'Cyclic corticosteroid immunosuppression is unsuccessful in the treatment of sperm antibody-related male infertility: a controlled study', *Human Reproduction*, vol 7 (1992), pp. 99–104.

190 Persson, J.W. et al, 'Is ICSI associated with risks of genetic disease? Implications for counselling, practice and research', *Human Reproduction*, vol 11 (1996), pp. 921–4.

191 Kurinczuk, J.J. and Bower, C., 'Birth defects in infants conceived by ICSI: an alternative interpretation', *British Medical Journal*, vol 315(7118) (1997), pp. 1260–66.

192 Fathalla, M.F., 'Incessant ovulation – a factor in ovarian neoplasia', *Lancet*, vol 1(ii) (1977), p. 163.

193 Stadel, B.V., 'The aetiology and prevention of ovarian cancer', *American Journal of Obstetrics and Gynaecology*, vol 123 (1975), pp. 772–4.

194 Shushan, A. et al, 'Human menopausal gonadotrophin and the risk of epithelial ovarian cancer', *Fertility and Sterility*, vol 65 (1996), pp. 13–8.

195 Potashnik, G., 'Fertility drugs and the risk of breast and ovarian cancers: result of a long-term follow-up study' *Fertility and Sterility*, vol 71(5) (1999) pp. 853–9.

196 The National Birthday Trust, 57 Lower Belgrave Street, London SW1.

197 Kadrabova, J. et al, 'Changed serum trace element profile in Down's syndrome', *Biological Trace Element Research*, vol 54(3) (1996), pp. 201–6.

198 *British Medical Journal*, vol 30 (1994), pp. 158–62.

199 Jennings, I., *Vitamins in Endocrine Metabolism*. William Heinemann, Medical Press (1972).

200 Regan, L., *Miscarriage*, Bloomsbury Publishing (1997).

201 Frisch, R.E., 'Food, intake, fatness and reproductive ability', in R.A. Vigersky (ed), *Anorexia nervosa*, Raven Press, New York (1977), pp. 139–61.

202 Regan, L., *Miscarriage*, Bloomsbury Publishing (1997).

203 Clark, A.M. et al, 'Weight loss in obese infertile women results in improvement in reproductive outcome for all forms of fertility treatment', *Human Reproduction*, vol 13(6) (1998), pp. 1502–5.

204 Stephens, N.G. et al, 'Randomised controlled trial of vitamin E in patients with coronary disease: Cambridge Heart Antioxidant Study (CHAOS)', *Lancet*, vol 347 (1996), pp. 781–6.

205 Furuhjelm et al, 'The quality of human semen in spontaneous abortion', *International Journal of Fertility*, vol 7 (1962), pp. 17–21.

206 Sorahan, T. et al, 'Childhood cancer and parental use of tobacco: deaths from 1971 to 1976', *British Journal of Cancer*, vol 76(11) (1997), pp. 1525–31.

207 Himmelberger, D.U. et al, 'Cigarette smoking during pregnancy and the occurrence of spontaneous abortion and congenital abnormality', *American Journal of Epidemiology*, vol 108 (1998), pp. 470–79.

208 Golding, Professor J., Royal Hospital for Children, Bristol, 'Talk given to a conference on Smoking in Pregnancy', commissioned by the Health Education Authority (1994).

209 Bennet, H.S. et al, 'Breast and prostate in men who die of cirrhosis of the liver', *American Journal of Clinical Pathology*, vol 20 (1950), pp. 814–28.
Kulikauskas, V. et al, 'Cigarette smoking and its possible effect on sperm', *Fertility and Sterility*, vol 44 (1985), pp. 526–8.

210 Kaufman, M., 'Alcohol threat to babies', *The Sunday Times* (31 January 1988).

211 Kline, J. et al, 'Smoking: A risk factor for spontaneous abortion', *New England Journal of Medicine*, vol 297 (1977), pp. 793–6.

212 Kline, J. et al, 'Drinking during pregnancy and spontaneous abortion', *Lancet*, vol 2 (1980), pp. 176–80.
Windham, G.C. et al, 'Moderate maternal alcohol consumption and risk of spontaneous abortion', *Epidemiology*, vol 5 (1997), pp. 509–14.

213 Zhang, H. and Bracken, M.B., 'Tree-based, two-stage risk factor analysis for spontaneous abortion', *American Journal of Epidemiology*, vol 144(10) (1996), pp. 989–96.

214 Furuhashi, N. et al, 'Effects of caffeine ingestion during pregnancy', *Gynecological and Obstetric Investigation*, vol 19 (1985), pp. 187–91.

Wichit, S. and Bracken, M.B., 'Caffeine consumption during pregnancy and association with late abortion', *American Journal of Obstetrics and Gynecology*, vol 154 91985), pp. 14–20.

215 Infante Rivard, C., *Journal of the American Medical Association* (22 December 1993).

216 Fenster, L. et al, 'A prospective study of caffeine consumption and spontaneous abortion', *American Journal of Epidemiology*, vol 143(11), 525, abstract no 99 (1996).

217 Barrington, J.W. et al, 'Selenium deficiency and miscarriage: a possible link?', *British Journal of Obstetrics and Gynaecology*, vol 103 (1996), pp. 130–2.

218 Bradley, B., *Preparation for Pregnancy*, Argyll Publishing (1995).

219 Webb, T., reported in Thomas Stuttaford, 'The screen of fear', *The Times* (15 November 1984).

220 Bramwell, R.S. and Davidson, M.J., 'Visual display units and pregnancy outcome: a prospective study', *Journal of Psychosomatic Obstetrics and Gynecology*, vol 14(3) (1993), pp. 197–210.

McDonald, A.D. et al, 'Visual display units and pregnancy: evidence from the Montreal survey', *Journal of Occupational Medicine*, vol 28(12), pp. 1226–31.

221 De Matteo, *The Terminal Shock*, NC Press, Toronto (1985).

222 Barnea, E.R. and Tal, J., 'Stress-related reproductive failure', *Journal of In Vitro Fertility, Embryo Transfer*, vol 8 (1991), pp. 15–23.

Wright, J. et al, 'Psychological distress and infertility, a review of controlled research', *International Journal of Fertility*, vol 134 (1989), p. 2.

223 Poston, L. et al, 'Effect of antioxidants on the occurrence of pre-eclampsia in women at increased risk: a randomised trial', *Lancet*, vol 354 (1999), pp. 810–19.

224 Williams, M.A. et al, 'Omega 3 fatty acids in maternal erythrocytes and risk of pre-eclampsia', *Epidemiology*, vol (3) (1995), pp. 232–7.

225 Stein, Z. et al, *Famine and Human Development*, Oxford University Press (1975).

226 Wynn, M. and Wynn, A., 'The importance of nutrition around conception in the prevention of handicap', *Applied Nutrition*, vol 1, British Dietetic Association (1981), pp. 12–19.

227 Wynn, M. and Wynn, A., *The Case for Preconception Care of Men and Women*, AB Academic, Bicester (1991).

228 Conference Review, *Nutrition and Health*, vol 8 (1992), pp. 45–55.

229 Barker, D.J.P. et al, 'Foetal and placental size and risk of hypertension in adult life', *British Medical Journal*, vol 301 (1990), pp. 259–62.

230 Barker, D.J.P. et al, 'Weight in infancy and death from coronary heart disease', *Lancet*, vol II (1989), pp. 577–80.

231 Hales, C.N. et al, 'Foetal and infant growth and impaired glucose tolerance at age 64', *British Medical Journal*, vol 303 (1991), pp. 1019–22.

232 Berankova, H., 'Maturity and fertility in women with low birthweights', *Casopia Lekaru Ceskych*, vol 136(13) (1997), pp. 413–15.

233 Jennings, I.W., *Vitamins in Endocrine Metabolism*, Heinemann (1970).

234 Library, The Royal College of Physicians (1725).

235 Smith, D.W., 'Alcohol effects in foetus' in 'Foetal Drug Syndrome: Effects of Ethanol and Hydantoins', *Paediatrics in Review 1*, American Academy of Paediatrics (1979).

236 Tuormaa, T., 'The Adverse Effects of Alcohol on Reproduction', *Journal of Nutritional and Environmental Medicine*, vol 6 (1996), pp. 379–91.

237 Streissguth, A.P., 'Foetal alcohol syndrome: an epidemiological perspective', *American Journal of Epidemiology*, vol 107 (1978), pp. 467–78.

238 Streissguth, A.P. et al, 'Neurobehavioral effects of prenatal alcohol; Part I, research strategy (Review of the literature)', *Neurotoxicology and Teratology*, vol 11 (1989), pp. 461–76.

239 Streissguth, A.P. et al, 'Moderate prenatal alcohol exposure: effects on child IQ and learning problems at age 7.5 years', *Alcohol Clinical Experimental Research*, vol 14 (1990), pp. 662–9.

240 Sullivan, J.F. and Lankford, H.G. 'Urinary excretion of zinc in chronic alcoholism', *American Journal of Clinical Pathology*, vol 45 (1962), pp. 156–9.

241 Flynn, A. et al, 'Zinc status of pregnant alcoholic women: A determination of foetal outcome', *Lancet* (14 March 1981), pp. 572–5.

242 Laurence, K.M. et al, 'Double-blind randomised controlled trial of folate treatment before conception to prevent recurrence of neural-tube defects', *British Medical Journal*, vol 282 (1981), pp. 1509–51.

243 Tuormaa, T., 'The adverse effects of tobacco smoking on reproduction and health: A review from the literature', *Nutrition and Health*, vol 10 (1995), pp. 105–20.

244 Ibid.

245 Carmichael, N.G. et al, 'Teratogenicity, toxicity and perinatal effects of cadmium', *Human Toxicology*, vol 1 (1982), pp. 159–86.

246 Health Education Authority leaflet.

247 Ibid.

248 Golding, Professor J., Talk given to a conference on Smoking in Pregnancy commissioned by the Health Education Authority (1994).

249 Schaefer, C. et al, 'Illnesses in infants born to women with Chlamydia trachomatis infection', *American Journal of Diseases of Children*, vol 139 (1985), pp. 127–33.
Sollecito, D., 'Prenatal Chlamydia trachomatis infection with postnatal respiratory disease in a preterm infant', *Acta Paediatri Scandinavia*, vol 76 (1987), p. 532.

250 Khattak, S., 'Pregnancy outcome following gestational exposure to organic solvents: a prospective controlled study', *Journal of the American Medical Association*, vol 281 (1999), pp. 1106–9.

251 Gerhard, I. et al, 'Toxic pollutants and fertility disorders: solvents and pesticides', *Geburtshilfe – Frauenheilkd*, vol 53(3) (1993), pp. 147–60.

252 Stenchever, M.A. et al, 'Chromosome breakages in users of marijuana', *American Journal of Obstetrics and Gynaecology*, vol 118 (1974), pp. 106–13.

253 Bongol, N. et al, 'Teratogenicity of cocaine in humans', *Journal of Pediatrics*, vol 1 (1987), pp. 93–6.

254 Ostrea, F.M. and Chavez, C.J., 'Perinatal problems (excluding neonatal withdrawal) in maternal drug addiction: a study of 830 cases', *Journal of Pediatrics*, vol 94 (1979), pp. 292–5.

255 Watanabe, G., 'Environmental determinants of birth defects prevalence', *Contributions to Epidemiology and Biostatistics*, vol 1, S. Karager, AG, Basel (1979), pp. 91–100.

256 Kocisova, J. et al, 'Mutagenicity studies on paracetamol in human volunteers: I Cytogenetic analysis of peripheral lymphocytes and lipid peroxidation in plasmas', *Mutation Research*, vol 209 (1988), pp. 161–5.

257 *Psychosomatics*, vol 30 (1989), pp. 25–31.

258 Yanai (ed), *Neurobehavioural Teratology*, Elsevier Science Publishers BV (1984).
The Initial Investigation and Management of the Infertile Couple, Evidence-Based Clinical Guidelines No 2, Royal College of Obstetricians and Gynaecologists (February 1998).

Recommended Reading

Miscarriage: What every woman needs to know by Professor Lesley Regan, Bloomsbury, 1997

Natural Fertility Awareness by John and Lucie Davidson, The CW Daniel Co., 1986

Fertility: Fertility awareness and natural family planning by Dr Elizabeth Clubb and Jane Knight, David & Charles, 1996

Preparation for Pregnancy by Suzanne Gail Bradley and Nicholas Bennett, Argyll Publishing, 1996

Planning for a Healthy Baby by Belinda Barnes and Suzanne Gail Bradley, Ebury Press, 1994

Silent Spring by Rachel Carson, Penguin Books, 1999

The Feminisation of Nature by Deborah Cadbury, Penguin Books, 1998

Our Stolen Future by Theo Colborn, Dianne Dumanoski and John Peterson Meyers, Abacus, 1997

Optimum Nutrition Cookbook by Patrick Holford, Piatkus Books, 1999

Superbug by Geoffrey Cannon, Virgin Publishing, 1996

How to Avoid GM Food by Joanna Blythman, Fourth Estate, 1999

Useful Addresses

Contacts

CHILD – The National Infertility Support Network
Charter House, 43 St Leonards Road, Bexhill-on-Sea, East Sussex TN40 1JA
Tel: 01424 732361

Healthy House (for natural paints, water filters, etc)
Cold Harbour, Ruscombe, Stroud, Glos GL6 6DA
Tel: 01453 752216

Human Fertilisation and Embryology Authority (HFEA)
Paxton House, 30 Artillery Lane, London E1 7LS
Tel: 020 7377 5077

ISSUE – The National Fertility Association
114 Lichfield Street, Walsall WS1 1SZ
Tel: 01922 722888

Miscarriage Association
Clayton Hospital, Northgate, Wakefield, West Yorks WF1 3JS
Tel: 01924 200799

National Endometriosis Society
50 Westminster Palace Gardens, Artillery Row, London SW1P 1RL
Tel: 020 7222 2781

Nutri Centre
7 Park Crescent, London W1B 1PF
Tel: 020 7436 5122

Premature Menopause Support Group
PO Box 392, High Wycombe, Bucks HP15 7SH

Quitline
A free helpline to encourage people to stop smoking. Has a Quitpack containing booklets, leaflets and information on the best way to stop smoking.
Tel: 0800 002200

Reproductive Healthcare
19 Cornwall Terrace, London NW1 4QP
Tel: 020 7935 7514

Toxoplasmosis Trust
61–71 Collier Street, London N1 9BE
Tel: 020 7713 0663

Verity – The Polycystic Self-Help Group
Trindlemanor, 52–54 Featherstone Street, London EC1Y 8RT

What Doctors Don't Tell You (monthly newsletter, sold by subscription – call for details)
2 Salisbury Road, London SW19 4EZ
Tel: 0870 444 9886

Complementary Medicine Organisations

Nutritional Therapy

British Association of Nutritional Therapists
BCM BANT, London WC1N 3XX
Tel: 0870 6061284

Acupuncture

The British Acupuncture Council
63 Jeddo Road, London W12 9HQ
Tel: 020 8735 0400

Homeopathy

Society of Homeopaths
4a Artizan Road, Northampton NN1 4HU
Tel: 01604 621400

Medical Herbalism

National Institute of Medical Herbalism
56 Longbrook Street, Exeter EX4 6AH
Tel: 01392 426022

Index

Staying in touch

If you have any health problems and are interested in finding a more natural approach to treating them or would like to find out what supplements and tests are available to you please feel free to contact me on the number below and I will send you more information on how you can help yourself.

Workshops, cassettes and videos

I give workshops and talks around the country and have produced cassettes and videos from some of these. Please call if you would like to find out more about future workshops and/or the recordings and you will be sent an information pack.

Consultations

If you want to see or talk to someone personally, I am available for private consultations at the following clinics, and postal consultations can be arranged: **The Hale Clinic, Regents Park, London** or **Women's Health-care, St John's Wood, London**

For appointments and enquiries:

Dr M Glenville the Nevill Estate, Danegate, Eridge Green, Tunbridge Wells, Kent TN3 9JA. Tel: 01892 750511 Fax: 01892 750533
Email: health@marilynglenville.com   www.marilynglenville.com

If you would like to hear more advice from Dr Marilyn Glenville on any of the following subjects:

- **Natural alternatives to Dieting** *How to lose weight naturally*
- **Natural alternatives to HRT** *How to stay healthy through the Menopause and prevent Osteoporosis*
- **Natural solutions to Infertility** *How to increase your chances of conceiving and preventing miscarriages*

Then call **0906 7010030** and select your choice for the information you would like to hear about.

Calls are charged at 50p per minute at all times. Helpline No: 01892 750511.

Also by Marilyn Glenville PhD

The Natural Health Handbook for Women
The ultimate reference guide for women of all ages

Everything you needed to know on the most effective ways to treat all aspects of your health naturally. In this important book, Dr Glenville guides you through a comprehensive list of female conditions and concerns. Throughout, she provides helpful insights and background information, compares and combines orthodox and natural treatments and provides reassuring advice on the most effective nutrition, supplements, herbs and tests for each health problem. Whether you suffer from fibroids, painful periods or endometriosis, or if you are going through a major life change such as pregnancy or the menopause, you'll learn how to help yourself in the most natural way possible. *The Natural Health Handbook for Women* offers understanding, and a comprehensive, safe and holistic approach. It is a must-have book for all women of all ages.

The Nutritional Health Handbook for Women
The book for every woman who cares about her health

The ultimate reference book for women of all ages. *The Nutritional Health Handbook for Women* tells you everything you need to know about the most effective ways to treat all aspects of your health naturally. Dr Marilyn Glenville believes that many female health problems are caused by incorrect nutrition and can be dramatically improved through simple changes to your diet and lifestyle. Based on 20 years of clinical experience and research, her approach is proven, highly successful and non-invasive.

Natural Solutions to PMS

Is Premenstrual Syndrome inevitable? Are women doomed to experience mood swings, weight gain, pain and discomfort each month throughout their reproductive life? In this book, Dr Marilyn Glenville, says emphatically, no. She explains there are simple nutritional and lifestyle changes you can make that will bring your hormones back into their natural balance and provide permanent relief for your symptoms. From breast pain to irritability, and from bloating to fatigue, Marilyn Glenville details a thoroughly researched and tested programme to get you feeling on top form every day of the month.